Welcome from Edita

This is my special letter to all those who have followed my health and nutritional program in my books and to all those who have lost weight and gained in health with me.

I want you to know, that I am and always was committed to bringing you the newest, the best, the most exciting programs to help you and those you love get healthier, get fitter, lose fat, and enjoy and protect the body that the good Lord blessed you with.

And that's why I never stop reading. Learning. Sharing with you. And that's why I welcome you to what I call the "prequel" to my Skinny System.

When I was first with the successful, and ground-breaking AM-PM Skinny System, which made losing as easy as telling time, by concentrating on fat blocking foods in the AM hours and switching to fat burning foods in the PM hours, much of the research in this book was not yet available. But now it is. And I'm delighted to once again, be the first to bring you this truly breakthrough diet and the research that inspired it.

You may ask, how *The Calcium Diet* fits with my *Skinny AM-PM Program*. Easy. *The Calcium Diet* is the prequel to your good health, longevity, and above all your success in the fight against fat.

I have maintained my commitment to the fat blocking AM foods and the fat burning PM foods that have resulted in such overwhelming weight loss successes for so many of you. But now, I have incorporated the newest research into weight loss and health and added it to my ongoing search for health and diet solutions. By adding nonfat dairy products, non-dairy foods high in calcium and/or calcium supplements *The Calcium Diet* enhances the programs I have previously developed—enhances them and takes them to new frontiers. But, whether you have been one of my "skinny stars" or whether you have followed other weight loss programs, you should be aware that adding dietary calcium to your daily diet may help you achieve your goals even more effectively and offer general health benefits besides.

God bless and keep you all.   *Edita*

How To Get In Touch With Edita

If you would like a personal consultation; if you are with the media and would like an interview; or if you would like to arrange for a speaking engagement for your company or organization; or if you would just like to say, "hello" you can reach me at my personal e-mail address EditaMKaye@aol.com

Lose 69% More Fat Now!

The Calcium Diet

The weight loss breakthrough spotlighting groundbreaking research into the super nutrient powers of calcium in successful, nutrition-based fat metabolism, weight loss, health & longevity

Easy-To-Follow 21-Day Calcium Diet!

PLUS 101 Recipes

By
Edita Kaye

Important Please Read Carefully

The information, ideas, suggestions, and answers to questions in this book are not intended to substitute for the services of a physician. You should only undertake a fat loss, weight loss, and health and wellness modification program in conjunction with the services of a qualified health professional. This book is intended as a reference guide only, not as a manual for self-treatment. If you suspect you have a medical problem or have questions, please talk to your health care professional. All the information here is based on research available at the time of this printing. All phone numbers, web addresses and references were current at the time of printing. Nutritional values are approximate. Information contained herein came from public sources.

Copyright 2003 The Calcium Research Institute
All rights reserved.
The Calcium Diet
830-13 A1A North,
Ponte Vedra Beach, FL 32082

www.thecalciumdiet.com or www.skinny.com

Printed in the United States of America
First Printing: October 2003

First Printing

ISBN 0-9740955-1-6

Library of Congress Cataloging-in-Publication Data
Kaye, Edita. 1. Weight loss. 2. Nutrition.

Dedication

*This book is dedicated
to the millions of American
men, women and children
who are fighting their own daily battle
with fat and the diseases of fat,
and to the researchers
who have dedicated themselves
to seeking out
the tools of victory.*

God bless and keep you all.

Other Books by Edita

Cooking Skinny With Edita
Skinny Rules
The Skinny Pill
The Fountain of Youth
Bone Builders Cookbook & Calcium Health Guide

Testimonials for *The Skinny Pill*

My gym had a contest to see who could make the most difference in their body over 3 months. I entered and then found *The Skinny Pill* to help me along and it really did help. I won second place out of 50 people. I started out at 144 and now I weigh 114. I even lost inches in my forearms and calves. Altogether I lost 30 pounds, 8.2% body fat and a total of 30 total inches, all in 3 months. Thanks! *Skinny Pill.*

Thank you. To date I have lost 20 pounds, 3-inches and 2 dress sizes! Could not have done it without *The Skinny Pill.*

…. Just to let you know it is for my mother-in-law. Since last May she has been following the book and taking the Skinny Pill and has lost 17 lbs! She looks really good and raves about how she is eating now more than ever!

I have lost over 50 pounds and have *The Skinny Pill* book…I do want you to know I have suggested it to many friends and they also have lots of results!

I weigh 232 lbs. I want to lose 80 lbs. I started the Skinny program and within one week lost 11 ¼ inches and 8 lbs. I heard about *The Skinny Pill* on the radio and I want to let you know how happy I am. People are already noticing my weight loss. I'm telling all my co-workers about how great the program is. I send you a big "thank you".

I have lost 12 pounds in 12 days following the plan. I do admit I have cheated a little on the weekends. But I follow your plan to the tee during the week. I forgot to measure myself. I can tell from the way my clothes fit I have lost inches. I'm hoping to be able to confirm more pounds and inches soon.

Hi, I lost 20 pounds in one-and-a-half months with strict adherence to *The Skinny Pill* plan. I haven't taken my "after" measurements but am down to size 11/12 instead of size 14.

Am going out of town for the weekend and had to buy a new outfit...I have lost two dress sizes in a bit over two weeks. I am amazed that this is working. Guess I will get leveled off at a point but I will keep going. Thanks so much!

Just wanted to let you know...on week 3 of *The Skinny Pill*...and I'm melting away. Already getting comments about how slim and trim I'm looking. I have no idea how much weight I've lost as I don't want to be tied to a scale. I just want to look good and feel great. Looking good and feeling great is a good option as well. The pill/program is working...along with that darn exercise. Thank you.

I have been on the Skinny Diet for 9 months and have lost 75 pounds.

I am happy to say that I have lost 72 pounds. I have only measured my hips and stomach and have lost a combination of 17 inches in those two areas. *The Skinny Pill* has really helped me and I have recommended it to so many people that I can't keep track. I am meeting up with my four sisters who are trying it…and can't wait to see how skinny they have all got! 15 more to go for me— yahoo!

Let me start off by saying that I'm female, 25 years old and have two young children. I have always had a problem with my weight. I never understood the problem until I read your book and realized that it was because I was either over eating the wrong foods or starving my body. I started your lifestyle (I say lifestyle because diets come and go and are fads, this is a way of life for me now) 2 weeks ago. I'm 5'9" and usually weighed anywhere from 240- 220. The day I started I weighed myself and weighed 221 and two weeks and one day later I weigh 205! I don't weigh everyday because I understand that daily weights are going to differ. I have gotten several compliments from co- workers and my own mother as to how much better I'm starting to look. I have energy now and don't feel drained at 6 p.m. every night. I can keep up with my kids who are 3 and 4 ½. I'm not only doing this for myself but for my two girls. I want to be healthy for them and have them not embarrassed of me when they start school. I just wanted to say thank you so much. You have changed my life in such a way that you will never totally understand. I tell everyone about you and your website now. Thank you.

My husband and I both went on the diet August 8, 2000. To date (September 12, 2000) we have both lost about 13 pounds. We are also seeing a difference in the fat build-up around our middles. We are very happy with the diet, and have recommended it to several people. But the biggest reason we began this diet was to find a way to naturally lower my blood pressure and cholesterol and triglycerides which I have not been able to be done with medicine due to allergies. I go back to my doctor on Oct. 10 at which time she will draw blood to see if those levels have changed due to this diet. She is also excited about the diet, has read the book (*The Skinny Pill*) and recommended it to several of her patients. Thank you.

Dear Edita: I actually bought *The Skinny Pill* for my friend. Since she has been taking it and watching what she eats, "Edita Style" she has lost a total of 35 pounds and has gone from a size eighteen to a size twelve. Unfortunately we didn't measure inches. But she is still losing weight and it is all thanks to you.

I've lost only 10 lbs but I've lost 23 inches in less than 4 months.

I have lost 55 pounds from January to July and have kept it off since. I have lost over 34 inches.

I love this way of eating. I'm never hungry and I feel I'm eating a more balanced diet. I have lost 10 pounds and 5 inches.

I have lost 29 pounds and 18 inches total.

I just wanted to thank you. My wife and I started on your plan on March 29, 2001. She has lost 11 lbs (as of May 11, 2001) and the light on the scale for normal weight (a person 5'3") started flashing yesterday morning. She went from 151 to 140. I started out at 250 and this morning I weighed in at 232.2 or 17.8 lbs less than 43 days ago. My goal is to get to 199. Actually my goal and my doctor's. How I got started. On March 23 I met a friend that I had not seen in a year and she at that time had lost 51 pounds. She told me about your plan and I went and bought your book. Again, thank you.

I am now up to 21 pounds lighter and my wife is at 11. Of course I have a lot more to give. People are starting to notice and I know of one person who went out and bought your book. Thanks for putting something together that I can live with.

I've been using the program for 2 weeks now. I have only lost about 6 lbs but I have lost 18 inches total. Thank you so much for this wonderful program.

Thank you. Fifteen pounds in one week. For the first time I have a positive attitude about a diet plan, and believe me I have tried them all. For the first few days I felt guilty about eating so often but not any more. Thank you again.

Thank you, thank you, thank you!!! I have only been taking the Skinny Pills for ONE week, and I've already lost 10 INCHES!!!! I have tried every diet known to woman over my lifetime and have probably lost more than 10,000 pounds. But, as I'm sure you know, I've put every one back on, plus a few more each time. And with each "diet" I had to give up all the things I love to eat. But not this time!! Just by taking your Skinny Pills and loosely following the Skinny Food Plan, I've finally found a way of eating that I can live with for the rest of my life!! And since I'm not giving anything up, I'm not going to be craving anything when I finally reach my desired weight, so I know THIS time I'll be able to maintain it. Thank you so much for giving me my life back, Edita!

I discovered your website and daily e-mail encouragements while trying to lose weight for my recent trip to Jamaica (just returned this weekend). Although I did not lose ALL of the weight I wanted to before my trip, I was able to lose HALF. Often your daily tips were what helped me get over each bump. I am not, per se, a heavy person—quite the opposite actually—I am in the need to tone more than anything, however, I am 41 and know that I am on an uphill climb of keeping my thin body. It's often hard to talk with my friends who are fighting their weight control more because I often receive "DIET?" Why? I WISH I was as thin." But see, I know it is in my genes to not be this size forever, so I must keep fighting it daily. You have helped, Edita, because with you I can receive advice without feeling bad! Thank you.

As I e-mailed you, my husband and I have lost so much weight on this diet (or as I like to call it—our life style program). I have been on every diet that has come out over the past many years. Some worked for awhile, some failed completely. This is the first program I have been very successful with—losing 75 pounds so far, and looking forward to losing 50 pounds more. My husband lost 55 pounds and is maintaining. This program fits into our lifestyle perfectly. Even my husband, who thought eating six times a day would be impossible, has found it works great. The morning and afternoon snacks he takes in the car with him, and he was able to eat out with customers, etc—sometimes they couldn't even tell he was dieting. We have shared this program with so many people. Many at the office where my husband works bought the book (*The Skinny Pill*) and wanted the same success as him. Many here at the Church where I work as Office Manager and also we attend the Church, have asked where to buy the book and many have gone on it. One of my secretaries started the program a couple of weeks ago, and has already had great success. Thanks so much! It is so fun to look back at pictures of ourselves from last year and say, "yeh—we sure can see a difference." More importantly, we feel so much better and my blood pressure is so much better and I have more energy than I have had for a long time!! Thanks again.

I have lost 21 pounds thus far on *The Skinny Pill* diet and I'm so pleased! It's been almost a month, I believe.

I have lost over 90 lbs and have never felt better. I have been on the program for over a year and a half.

Hi…I started on the program this Monday. Today is the start of day 5 and believe it or not I have lost 15 pounds. I have two different scales at home and both indicate that I've lost 15 pounds. I could not believe it. I do not feel deprived on the menu, in fact I feel as though I am eating more food than I normally do. I have been dieting for over 12 years with no success. I could not lose any weight and keep it off. For one thing I have Hashimoto's disease—my thyroid does not function and I am on thyroid medication. I've been to so many doctors and have tried every diet in the world and every supplement and shakes and power bars but none have worked. I was getting so discouraged since I have gained over 100 lbs in the past two years. I hate the way I look in clothes and I see people staring at me and thinking that I must eat like a pig. I exercise regularly and I have been watching what I eat but nothing has worked like your program. I am so thrilled that I found out about *The Skinny Pill* and I want to share it with every overweight person out there. I know that this is the program that I can stick with.

Let's see to begin with I would like to lose about 80 lbs. I began the program nine days ago and weighed 229.5. I checked in this morning at 223.5. Needless to say I think I'm off to a good start.

Dear Edita. My manicurist showed me the magazine with your diet in it. She had been on it for about a week and had lost 5 pounds so I ran out and got a copy and both my husband and I are on the diet and are in our second week. I have lost 9 ½ pounds and 1 ½ inches around my waist (I'm afraid to measure those fat hips so quickly) and he has lost 7 pounds.

Hello. I ordered your Skinny Pills and book a number of months ago. I didn't have a ton of weight to lose but I was having a hard time losing what I wanted to. Your book really showed me "how" to eat. I was eating a lot of extra food that I didn't need. I have encouraged friends and family members to try it out as well. My aunt and her husband recently purchased it from my referral. I lost 10 pounds in the first 14 days. The diet to follow is really worth it!

Thank you. Thank you. Thank you. It's been 9 days now. My wife and I went to an anniversary party last night and the first person who saw me called me over and asked how much I had lost. I am not able to weight myself on a regular scale yet (our scale registers at 330 lbs) but I think I've lost around 20 lbs. My clothes are starting to hang and I feel great. My goal is 225. I'm on my way. My wife is having fun trying on the "small clothes" too. Thanks again!

Thank you so much for the daily weight loss advice. I have kept off 25 pounds and have started walking again.

Hi Edita. Just wanted to wish you a very happy birthday and to tell you thank you for all you have done. I have tried so many programs and bought so many books and finally this is the one that is working for me. It is fun and easy and I love the emails. God bless and thanks again.

Happy birthday, Edita. I love this diet. I have lost about 10 pounds in a month (started at145 and down to 135). I have about 5-7 more pounds to go to reach my goal weight! I love this diet because I don't feel deprived and I love ice cream so I have a skinny sundae daily using frozen fat free chocolate yogurt! I love fat free frozen yogurt now!!! My doctor thought it sounded like a good diet as well!! My friends have asked about it and have told me I am getting "skinny"! which is a great incentive to keep on track. Thank you for taking the time and energy to research this diet and create it to help people like me who have such a hard time losing weight. I say this because I am "hypothyroid" which makes it very difficult for me to lose weight! I finally found what works for me. The other thing that is really hard is I own my own business. I work with delicious chocolates and candies from all over the world all day long and have not had a craving to eat them since I have been on this diet. My husband who is very skeptical of all diets and needs to lose about 30 pounds himself has been impressed with the amount of food I can eat and what I eat and still I am able to lose weight. (I'm hoping he'll go on this diet soon) My son lost 23 lbs in about 3 weeks also on this diet. He is a big football player who weighed about 315 and needs to lose quite a bit of weight. Thank you so much, Edita.

Bone Builder's Cookbook & Calcium Health Guide

This is my second book about calcium. My first book, *Bone Builders Cookbook* was written in 1995 and subsequently published by Warner Books. It was also a selection of the *Double Day Book Club.*

The preface to *Bone Builders* was written by Hugh R.K. Barber, M.D. He was at that time Professor of Clinical Obstetrics & Gynecology at Cornell University Medical College, New York; Director, Department of Obstetrics & Gynecology at Lenox Hill Hospital, New York, and Editor, *Female Patient Journal.* Here is what Dr. Barber had to say about my first calcium book, *Bone Builders.* I am very proud of my work in this first book and proud to share his comments and praise with you.

"This book is truly the ABC of the many contributions that calcium makes to a variety of organs and to maintaining a lifestyle that is marked by good health and longevity.

It is a book that should be read in its entirety. There may be a tendency to skip over the first part to get to the outstanding number of low fat, calcium-rich recipes but this would deny the reader an extensive understanding of the metabolic and physiologic mechanisms of calcium. This is more—namely, it is a reference book to which a physician or health care provider can turn as he or she searches for an answer about calcium.

It is not an overstatement to say that it is a book that supplies all you need to know about calcium. The purpose of this book is not to take the place of standard textbooks but to serve as an extension of the material found in those textbooks. It covers many facets of calcium without diluting the individual topic. It is structured so that the busy clinician, who shares the major burden of patient care, can keep abreast of the wide applications of calcium therapy for improving the health care of patients. The aim of the book is to present the basic and practical aspects of calcium in a readable format.

Edita M. Kaye has made the material in the book concise without being superficial and it will serve as an overall framework in which new knowledge will be placed and then used in the delivery of health care to women.

The author has borrowed freely from the literature and had included outstanding research and a credible bibliography. In addition, she has achieved simplicity of style, brevity, and clarity.

The author discusses the role of osteoporosis and cancer in the health care of women and does emphasize that the role of calcium affects all disciplines of medicine. She repeatedly states with documentation that calcium should be added as a supplement very early in life. It protects against many diseases and by doing this can bring the person into the menopause with an excellent bone mass, providing protection against those conditions that can be a bone robber.

The different parts of the book are well arranged and it leads from the beginning, getting to know calcium, on up through how new calcium research can help, provides ways of telling whether you're getting enough calcium and the signs and symptoms if there is a calcium deficiency. From time to time, the author presents a quiz that is well designed and adds a new dimension to the presentation.

In a very concise but accurate way, the author presents diagnostic wonders and what can be done immediately to correct bone loss. With courage, she even takes a peek into the future and does this in a very easy but readable manner.

She constantly points out what food substances can block the absorption of calcium and often provides ways to circumvent this. She accurately presents material on the fetus and calcium, what the requirements are, and how they can best be obtained.

Edita M. Kaye has presented material supporting the use of nutrients as a supplement to calcium therapy. There are many surprises for the health care provider in the presentation when she discusses potassium, magnesium, zinc, vitamin D, vitamin C and other supplements with charts giving the recommended daily allowances.

When she discusses calcium supplements, she accurately reports that the faster they dissolve the better the body absorbs them and she says that to test your own supplement all that is necessary is to drop one of the supplements into a glass of vinegar. If it hasn't dissolved after 30 minutes, it isn't being absorbed fast enough.

When discussing exercise, she has a pithy heading, which says, "Use It Or Lose It".

Her material on lactose intolerance and allergies is well presented.

The part of the book called the "The Nutrition Part" is excellent. She discusses the calcium in foods and presents it in a readable format. She has tips for identifying the value of milk, storing and handling it, as well as ways to structure breakfast, lunch, dinner and snacks so as to provide the best possible lifestyle. There is one section entitled "Add A Little Yogurt To Your Life" and she outlines how to do this. She also states and gives the reference that yogurt eaters have 25% fewer colds and that yogurt may boost the immune system by aiding in the production of gamma interferon.

Constantly there are one-liners that are truly medical pearls and add to the joy of reading this interesting presentation.

The last part is entitled "The Cookbook." It is fascinating that there are more than 150 low fat calcium recipes and many of them have a little editorial pearl at the end of the recipe. For example, in the recipe "Pineapple Carrot Raisin Muffins" there is a pearl that states that "Studies show that calcium is an antioxidant. Add the 20,000 IU of beta-carotene from carrots in this recipe and you have major protection from premature aging and disease." At the end of one recipe she states that the two minerals most deficient in American women's diets are calcium and iron. At the end of another, she states that calcium boosts brain power. This whole section is enriched by medical pearls. Having read through all of the recipes, one's appetite is stirred to the point where plans are made to try them one after another.

The book should be of interest to all health care workers, including medical students, residents, postgraduate fellows, physicians in practice and the general public which has so much interest in subjects relating to medicine. The lay public will find that it has brought the science of calcium together in one book for the benefit of the patient and at the same time it has been able to lighten the work of the busy physician.

The book qualifies as an outline for each physician's continuing medical education. Every aspect of the book is a plus and the only negative may be that it should have been written at least 15 years ago."

The Award Winning
Skinny Rules Book

From *The Midwest Book Review* "A disclaimer in Edita's *Skinny Rules* warns that its information is not a substitute for the services of a physician in devising a personal weight loss and fitness plan for a better, healthier life. With that caution firmly in mind, Edita's *Skinny Rules* is a wonderful supplement to professional guidance and filled cover to cover with tips, tricks, and techniques to putting one's psychology to work eating lighter and better and craving less, avoiding the impulse to eat out of boredom or appetite rather than real hunger, and dispensing myths about obesity. Accessibly written for the non-specialist general readers of all weights and backgrounds, Edita's *Skinny Rules* is an excellent addition to the serious dieter's reference shelf."

Table of Contents

Part Four   The Recipes Part   **164**

FAT BLOCKER Lunches (AM)

FAT BURNER Lunches (PM)

How To Benefit From This Book

How much can you lose? How fast can you lose? How easy is it going to be? Here's a sneak preview.

Studies show that just by being on any diet that restricts calories, you can expect to lose about 8% of your body fat and up to 11% of your body weight. Now look what happens when you add calcium. You can increase your weight loss by 25% and your fat loss by a whopping 69%!

That means that whatever diet you are on—*The Calcium Diet* can help you improve your results by up to 25%! What does this mean in real numbers? O.K. ladies, if you weigh 160 pounds and you have a decrease of 25% in body weight—that's 40 pounds. Guess what? Now you weigh 120 pounds! Men. If you weigh 220 pounds and you have a decrease of 25% in body weight—that's 55 pounds. Now you weigh 165 pounds! Do your own math on your own weight.

That means that *The Calcium Diet* alone can help you lose up to 25% more weight than you would on any other program and up to 69% more body fat than you would on any other program.

That's what makes *The Calcium Diet* so incredibly special and unique. Use it as your only diet. Add it to your favorite diet. Either way, you lose more fat and more weight than ever before. You can lose up to 25% more weight and up to 69% more fat with calcium.

What does that mean? Less body fat. A leaner shape. Lose up to 69% more fat from your tummy. From your waist. Lose up to 69% more fat from your thighs. From your back. Lose up to 69% more fat from your entire body and be rewarded with improved health, more energy, a reduced risk of fat-linked diseases, and the vanity factor of just plain looking and feeling better!

How fast? Studies now show that just by adding the equivalent calcium found in one glass of milk—300 mg you start to lose as much as six pounds, now! Add the calcium of 2 glasses of milk and that becomes 12 pounds! Keep it going!

Simple. Effective. Powerful. And the subject of dozens of new studies, reports, and experiments.

Welcome to America's newest, most exciting and promising, breakthrough diet featuring calcium information so new and so compelling based on scientific American studies, showing calcium can assist you not only in reaching your personal weight and fat loss goals, but can positively impact your health and longevity by reducing the risks for many life-threatening diseases.

But you don't have to take my word for it. Research this for yourself. See what the excitement is all about.

Now, about *The Calcium Diet*, itself. This is a diet based on the addition of a key dietary nutrient whose fat loss properties are the focus of some of the most innovative research from some of the most prestigious University research centers in the country.

This is a diet based on the addition of a key dietary nutrient linked with weight loss and improved health—a link that is currently taken seriously enough to be the subject of a government study.

This is a diet based on the addition of a key dietary nutrient, so important, without it America may enter deeper and deeper into the epidemic of obesity and without it researchers suspect that America will grow fatter and fatter, sicker and sicker, with heart disease, cancers, diabetes and more of the life-shortening, crippling and expensive results of obesity.

This is a diet based on the addition of a key dietary nutrient that could help reverse the epidemic of fat that threatens us and our children and that could enhance our health, increase our longevity, and help restore our lean and fit bodies.

What is this simple nutrient? What is this miraculous ingredient?

Simple. It's calcium. Better yet. It's milk. It's yogurt. It's cheese. It's vegetables. It's fish. It's food the good Lord created. It's supplements available everywhere.

This is the story of *The Calcium Diet*. How it began. What it can do. And how it can help you. How it can help those you love. It is a story that is just beginning. And you are in at the start.

The Calcium Diet is the continuing journey I have taken in researching and bringing you the cutting edge in health, wellness, nutrition, and weight loss.

The Calcium Diet brings me back, full circle to my first book, *Bone Builders*. Writing a few years ago, about calcium, there were just the tiniest of hints about the effect of this miraculous mineral on weight loss. Just whispers. Just fragile bubbles of hope. And so I waited. And watched. And read. And, like all of you, I hoped. And now my waiting, my research, my hope and yours, has been realized. It's still early days. A lot has still to be learned. To be understood. To be explored. But we have come a long way already. Ten years worth of academic research shows great promise and just a few months ago, the research into the powerful effects of calcium—specifically dairy-derived calcium—has prompted a two-year federal study.

The Buzz Begins: Highlights

The question being asked in government, medical, and media circles today is one that has created an almost unprecedented level of excitement. The question being asked is this, "Is there a single nutrient that can help lose weight?" And the excitement is due to what seems to be the answer to our most pressing health problem, obesity. Yes. The answer seems to be a resounding "yes."

The nutrient that has caused, and continues to cause the buzz, the excitement, the hope and the increasing research, is simply, calcium.

Is it possible, ask the scientists that America's epidemic of obesity is in part due to the fact that Americans get less than the recommended daily allowance of calcium? And is it possible that calcium can reverse the seemingly irreversible upward spiral of obesity?

- Are we getting fatter and fatter from too little calcium?
- Can we get thinner and thinner from more calcium?

Preliminary results are promising. And what do they promise? That perhaps the secret to shedding our fat is just a glass of milk away—

University Research Links Calcium & Fat Loss

University studies began to hit the media. Reports that Purdue University in Indiana researchers had discovered the calcium/weight loss connection during a study of the effect of exercise on bone mineral density in young women. The study found that regardless of how active they were—how much exercise they did—the young women who consumed the most calcium lost more body fat than those who were calcium deficient. The results were best in those women who ate a calorie-wise diet of no more than 1800 calories per day and who took the recommended daily calcium allowance of 1,000 mg. The Purdue researchers went on to find that women who took 780 mg of calcium stayed at the same body fat level while women who took less than 780 mg of calcium per day gained weight.

Creighton University in Omaha researchers examined the health records of hundreds of women and found that those who had the highest calcium intakes did not gain weight, while those with the lowest calcium intakes, did gain weight. Additionally it was found that those with the lowest calcium intake had the highest body fat levels.

The University of Utah reported findings of a study that showed children between the ages of four and eight who had their diets supplemented with more calcium and protein from dairy foods did not gain as much body fat as children who did not get the additional calcium nutritional support.

The University of Tennessee undertook to examine the diets of thousands of participants in a US food consumption study and found that women who consumed the most calcium, about 1,300 mg per day, were less likely to be obese than women who consumed fewer than 1,300 mg of calcium per day. By way of explanation, the researchers at the University of Tennessee suggested that low calcium levels seem to do two things that are fat and weight related. Low levels of calcium trigger a rise in the hormone parathyroid and also raise the levels of vitamin D. The hormone, parathyroid together with vitamin D work to regulate the absorption of calcium from the intestines and its movement in and out of bone tissue. But, and this is the key, one of the side-effects of these two, the hormone parathyroid and vitamin D is that if their levels are raised, there is a resulting accumulation of fat in fat cells. The result, more body fat. By the same token, increasing calcium levels signals other hormones that cause fat cells to release stored fat. Scientists warn that calcium plays an important role in metabolic disorders linked to obesity and insulin resistance, and higher levels of calcium seem to have a positive effect, reversing stored fat and releasing it. The results are beneficial with or without additional exercise, but are viable only at diets below a certain daily caloric intake—1800 or 1900 calories per day. Researchers are quick to point out, that this preliminary research should not send America to the couch—but that a daily exercise program, combined with a sensible low calorie diet, and additional calcium can have promising benefits in terms of body fat loss.

But the excitement is real. Study after study now shows that calcium is a powerful fat fighter.

Prevention reported that overweight people who took a calcium supplement lost 26% more body weight and 38% more body fat than those who ate the same calorie restricted diet minus the supplement. Another group, which got their calcium from dairy food sources lost 70% more weight and 64% more fat on a high-dairy diet that was low in calories, but that included three or four servings of low fat dairy products, totaling about 1,200 to 1,300 mg of calcium, per day. Much of the fat loss occurred in the belly area—an area which medical experts now believe to be a major risk factor for obesity-related diseases.

Explaining the research, investigators found that low levels of calcium appear to turn on a gene that tells cells to make more fat and inhibit fat breakdown. Boosting calcium to about 1,000 mg per day enhances weight loss. Cited was a recent study in which mice were divided into two groups. Both groups were put on the same restricted calorie diet. Group 1 received the human female equivalent of what average American women consume—500 mg of calcium per day. This group lost 8% of their body fat. Group II of the mice received a human calcium equivalent of 1,600 mg per day and lost 42 percent of their body fat. When the calcium was derived from dairy products the fat loss went up to 60 percent and more.

Reporting on past studies from the Nutrition Institute at the University of Tennessee, a researcher explained that three or four servings of low fat dairy products can help adjust the body's fat-burning machine and that low fat calcium may help reduce body fat. The studies seemed to show that the more calcium there is in a fat cell, the more fat it will burn—a higher calcium diet favors fat burning.

The research was promising. Mice were first fed a high fat/high sugar diet.

Next, the mice were divided into four groups.

Group I was placed on a calorie restricted diet alone. This group lost 8% in body fat.

Group II was placed on the same calorie restricted diet and were also given a calcium supplement. This group had a 42% decrease in body fat.

Group III was placed on the same calorie restricted diet and were also given calcium, through medium dairy. This group had a 60% decrease in body fat.

Group IV was placed on the same calorie restricted diet and were also given calcium, through a high dairy diet. This group had a 69% decrease in body fat.

This research was then translated and applied to human equivalents through the National Health and Nutrition Examination Survey (NHANES III) and confirmed that 3 eight-ounce glasses of skim milk could have major impact on fat and weight loss.

The National Institutes of Health, Center for Human Nutrition announced that, "Research indicates that higher levels of calcium in a controlled eating plan can help promote weight loss and leanness."

And in an article published in the *Journal of the American College of Nutrition* it was confirmed that each daily intake of 300 mg of calcium (about 8 ounces of milk) was associated with about six pounds lower weight in adults.

The calcium amounts in the study are effectively equal to what the USDA already recommends for adults.

The lead researchers from Creighton University, comment in a report that, "Data from six observational studies and three controlled trials...have been reanalyzed to evaluate the effect of calcium intake on body weight and body fat...taken together these data suggest that increasing calcium intake by the equivalent of two dairy servings per day could reduce the risk of overweight substantially, perhaps by as much as 70 percent."

And so I have taken what we know already. I have taken the promising results of this innovative, exciting, and life giving research and I present it here to you. I urge you to read carefully. To go beyond this book. To read the studies for yourself. To learn. To educate yourself. Because it is only through understanding, education, your commitment to living a long, healthy, and slender life, that you can achieve that goal for yourself. For now, I am only your guide. So, come, let's take the first steps together until you can walk alone—tall, strong, healthy, slim and vigorous.

The Calcium Diet is committed to education. It is an education about obesity, about calcium, about the latest research and about how you and the ones you love can benefit. There are no promises in this book. The only promise is the one you must make to yourself—to read—to learn—to use what you have read and learned for yourself.

Part One—The Fat Part is a real look at obesity in America and what it costs us, Americans, in health, wealth, and unhappiness. I urge you to read it. It is not pretty. In fact, it is terrifying. It is a look into our future if we don't begin—each one of us, individually—to take control over our own bodies. How? The same way we lost control—with a knife and a fork and a spoon—one mouthful at a time.

Part Two—The Calcium Part. Here is the necessary background into the miracle mineral we call calcium. Here you will read the excitement and urgency that surrounds this single nutrient from medical and government sources both—united in a common mission—to increase the level of awareness of calcium nutrition in America and among Americans, from the youngest, to the most senior. It outlines the increasingly important role calcium plays, not only as one of the newest recognized tools in our fight against obesity, but as a critical component in our overall health.

   Part Three—The Diet Part. It begins with the research currently available and goes on to show how this research can apply to you and then offers a 21-day Diet Plan designed just for you with both exercise and a personal journal. But there's more. There's a special diet section for people who just can't tolerate or just plain don't like dairy products, so they can get more calcium benefits from other foods. *The Calcium Diet* can be the only diet you'll ever need. But, I've included a very special section that shows you how to use the power of the Calcium Diet to enhance any diet program. *The Calcium Diet* is the perfect COMBO diet working to boost the power of your favorite diet program from Atkins to the Zone and everything in between.

   Part Four—The Recipes Part. Here are fabulous, delicious recipes to share with your family and friends and enjoy while you lose with every bite. The recipes are fast, simple and designed to fit into your busy life.

   Part Five—The Resources Part. Here are all the resources you'll need to use, lose and enjoy the health benefits of *The Calcium Diet* for life and living! Here is where you'll find food lists, shopping lists, tips on getting more calcium into your day, organizations to help you, and research sources to pursue on your own.

> *God bless you and yours.*
> *Edita Kaye*
> *Florida 2003*

Part One

The Fat Part

Chapter 1   How Fat Are We?

It seems all we have to do is look around our office, the food court in our mall, our grocery store, the Sunday morning brunch buffet at our favorite restaurant, the ticket line at the movie theatre, our own dining room table, or the mirror, to see the growing problem of fat in America.

The Media Reports Trends

On February 7, 2003 a *USA Today* headline announced, "Obesity rate could reach nearly 40% in five years." The article warned "nearly four out of 10 adults in the USA will be obese within five years if people keep packing on pounds at the current rate—putting their health at risk."

The article went on to offer shocking statistics to support the headline: 31% or 59 million people are obese, defined as roughly 30 or more pounds over a healthy weight. Almost 65% are either obese or overweight—10 to 30 pounds over a healthy weight. And Americans are gaining one to two pounds a year according to researchers at the Center for Human Nutrition at the University of Colorado Health Sciences Center.

The Government "Weighs In"

Date from media, medical and government sources highlights an alarming trend. No question. America is fat and getting fatter.

There's more. The National Health and Nutrition Examination Survey (NHANES) 1999 estimated 61 percent of U.S. adults are either overweight or obese, defined as having a body mass index (BMI) of 25 or more.

The National Center for Chronic Disease Prevention and Health Promotion reports that among U.S. adults aged 20-74 years, the prevalence of overweight (defined as BMI 25.0-29.9) has increased and that in the same population, obesity (defined as BMI greater than or equal to 30.0) has nearly doubled from approximately 15% in 1980 to an estimated 27% in 1999.

The result? Experts agree that the rise in obesity puts Americans at risk for developing diabetes, heart disease, some types of cancer and many other obesity-related health problems or health problems suspected of being linked to obesity.

The Medical Community Concurs

The Journal of the American Medical Association in 1999 reported obesity rates increased from 12% in 1991 to 17.9% in 1998. This was a steady increase occurring in all states; in both sexes; across all age groups, races, education levels; and occurred whether or not a person smoked.

Fat Dollars At Work

But beyond the cost to our health and quality of life, obesity is expensive.

A two-year study of 200,000 workers at a major corporation, designed to examine the relationship between medical costs and the six weight groups as outlined in the U.S. National Heart, Lung, and Blood Institute's weight guidelines reported in the *American Journal of Health Promotion* (January/February 2003) that the average annual medical costs for people with normal weight was $2,225 while the average annual medical costs for people who were overweight were $2,388 and $3,753 for people who were obese. The study also found that 40 percent of the workers were overweight. And that's just one company.

The national costs are staggering. The U.S. Department of Health and Human Services reports that in 2000 the total economic costs to the nation associated with obesity were $117 billion!

Mature Americans And Fat

A study conducted by the federal Centers for Disease Control found that obesity is a growing problem for older Americans. In the past 10 years, Americans between 60 and 70 years of age experienced the highest increase in obesity of any age group in the U.S.

Fat And Our Children and Grandchildren

And let's not forget our children. Here are truly frightening statistics.

On March 13, 2002, Howell Wechsler, Ed.D., M.P.H. Health Scientist, Division of Adolescent and School Health CDC's National Center for Chronic Disease Prevention and Health Promotion, testified before the Maryland Senate Education Committee on the Trends in Dietary Behaviors and Overweight Among Young People.

This distinguished scientist reported, "Between 1980 and 1999 the prevalence of overweight among children nearly doubled and, among adolescents, it nearly tripled."

He went on to express grave concern, about this increase in overweight among children and adolescents pointing out that studies have shown overweight children are at increased risk for the physiological risk factors such as elevated cholesterol levels, high levels of insulin, high blood pressure and more, that can lead to cardiovascular disease and diabetes.

He also pointed to the disturbing increase in type 2-diabetes among our children. The form of diabetes known as type-2 diabetes or "adult onset diabetes" because it typically occurs in the middle adult years was now increasingly found in children. In fact it was in 1979 that the first case of an adolescent diagnosed with type-2 diabetes was ever reported in a medical journal. That's not the case today. Today, diabetes clinics across the nation are reporting many such cases. Between 8 percent and 45 percent of recently diagnosed cases of diabetes among children and adolescents in the U.S. is adult onset diabetes, and the magnitude of this disease may be underestimated. He goes on to warn that, "Type-2 diabetes among youth may be the first consequence of the epidemic of obesity observed among North American youth."

So the fat crisis in America is universal. It involves us. It involves our parents. And most tragically, it involves our children and our grandchildren.

Chapter 2   How Did We Get So Fat?

Theories abound. And the only positive note on the whole fat landscape, is that we ourselves are not entirely to blame for our out-of-control fat situation. In fact the one consistent note seems to be that there is not one single reason, but many reasons, that we are now floating on an ocean of fat, and heading right for the obesity equivalent of the perfect storm.

Sugar

While we have been dutifully buying lower fat foods for over a decade, it may well be, that one of the biggest reasons we are getting fatter is not dietary fat at all, but sugar.

According to the USDA, the average American consumes about 20 teaspoons of sugar per day. The Center for Science in the Public Interest reports "added sugars—found largely in junk foods such as soft drinks, cakes, and cookies—squeeze healthier foods out of the diet." It makes a very sobering display, to measure out 20 teaspoons of sugar—that's almost one-half cup every single day!

In a letter to the Secretaries of the U.S. Department of Health and Human Services (HHS) and the U.S. Department of Agriculture (USDA) over forty health and nutrition experts called for a National Academy of Sciences (NAS) study on the health consequences of sugar consumption citing medical evidence indicating that diets high in sugar can promote obesity, kidney stones, osteoporosis, heart disease and dental caries.

The experts added, "That sugar now accounts for 16 percent of the calories consumed by the average American and 20 percent of teenagers' calories." This is a disturbing increase based on a government study that found that in 1977-1978 added sugars provided only 11 percent of the average person's calories.

The finger of sugar blame points primarily to soft drinks which contain about nine teaspoons of sugar per 12-ounce can and to the fact that per capita consumption of soda has doubled since 1974.

Where is all this sugar coming from? The soft drink risk is increasingly evident among children. Studies now link increased obesity to sugar intake, especially in sodas. A study conducted by the Harvard School of Public Health that tracked 548 ethnically diverse 11-to-12-year-old children over a two-year period found that the odds of becoming obese increased 1.6 times for each additional can or glass of soft drink consumed each day compared to baseline consumption of 1 can or glass per day.

More evidence piles on. In 1994 the Continuing Survey of Food Intakes by Individuals (CSFII) found that children between the ages of 2 and 18 who consumed soft drinks also consumed an average of 2018 calories per day compared to 1830 calories per day for those children who did not consume soft drinks. Do the math. Kids who drink sodas consumed an extra 188 calories per day. That's a whole pound (3500 calories) in 18.6 days!

And the studies continue.

Genetics

Howard Hughes Medical Institute at Rockefeller University opines that basic differences in individual's genetics may play a role in both obesity and the ability to retain slenderness despite the growing epidemic of obesity.

The genetic riddle is being examined on a number of different research fronts: sets of genes which are part of a physiological system designed to maintain weight consistency in individuals. Hormones, such as leptin, may hold the key to genetic management of rampant obesity.

Environment

This is a category that includes an assortment of factors, from lack of exercise, to television viewing, to suburban development and the automobile, even to outdoor temperature variations.

According to the Georgia Division of Public Health, the more likely reason for the increase in obesity in the Southern States, as compared to the New England and Western States, is the lack of exercise and the fact that Southerners are less likely to hike, ride a bike, walk or join a health club than their counterparts in the rest of the nation. Could it be the heat? Possibly.

But whether climate is a culprit or not, many communities are not conducive to walking. Cars are the major form of transportation, even to the corner store. It even goes beyond simple walking. Most of us select the elevator, even for a short trip of one or two flights, when the stairs would provide a healthier alternative.

Portion Sizes

Here it comes. Portions are also blamed. *The Journal of the American Dietetic Association* reports a steady increase in portion sizes over time. And a study in the *Journal of the American Medical Association* found that between 1977 and 1998 nearly all food portions increased both at home and in restaurants. The study points out that during that time period, the serving size of an average soft drink increased from 13 ounces and 144 calories to nearly 20 fluid ounces and 193 calories. The average cheeseburger grew from 5.8 ounces to 7.3 ounces and from 397 calories to 533 calories.

And the sizes of many products are also larger today than when they first appeared on the consumer market. For example, a regular sized fountain soda served at one fast food outlet in 1954 is now equivalent to today's child-size drink. The original regular soda at another fast food outlet was five ounces smaller than the current child size portion served in today's outlets.

Advertising

In a report in *Diabetes Care* in 2003, a researcher examined 2001 U.S. spending on fast food advertising by brand via print, television, radio and other media. Advertising for fast food alone, amounted to $3.5 billion, with an additional $5.8 billion spent on advertising for foods, confections and beverages, of which an astounding $786 million was spent for the top five brands of soda. This, compared to the total budget of the CDC for the same year of $5 billion. And the U.S. Food and Drug Administration budget of just $1.3 billion. Powerful media messages may well be a contributing factor to the increase in American obesity. There is just so much more money advertising "junk food" than there is advertising good nutritional health.

Confusion

Challenges to our long-health nutritional beliefs are also popping up as reasons for America's increase in obesity and seeming inability to fight the tide of fat.

Recently, critics have begun to lay blame on the rise in obesity on some of our most widely held beliefs about healthy nutrition.

A press release issued by Simon & Schuster, publishers of *The Harvard Medical School Guide to Healthy Eating* promoting the new title, claims, "The USDA Food Pyramid is wrong"

The author of the book, Walter C. Willett, M.D., one of the world's most distinguished experts in nutrition, reveals the danger behind this deceptive resource and provides a new pyramid that offers potential for longer, and better, living. Derived from decades of research based on the world-famous Harvard Nurses' Health Study, the Harvard Physicians Health Study, and Health Professionals Follow-up Study, the Framingham Heart Study and supported by dozens of other surveys and investigations…at best, the author claims that the USDA Pyramid offers indecisive, scientifically unfounded advice on absolutely a vital topic—what to eat. At worst, the misinformation it offers contributes to overweight, poor health, and unnecessarily early deaths."

There's more controversy brewing. A recent article in the March/April 2003 issue of *Modern Maturity*, the Journal of the American Association of Retired Persons—a powerful and large organization—as part of a feature on obesity and seniors, reports, " Along with being constantly tempted by food, we've also been given bad—or at least incomplete—advice from the very people we trusted to tell us how to eat; the U.S. government and the nation's largest and most respected health organizations." The article goes on to explain, "For decades, Americans were told that the primary cause of weight gain was eating fatty, greasy foods. A healthy diet, according to the federal government, the American Heart Association, and others was heavy in carbohydrates—the rice, bread, cereals, and pasta that form the wide base of the government's much-touted "food pyramid". Fresh fruits and vegetables come next in the pyramid, then meat and dairy, and then most sparingly, fats and oils." The article concedes "At the time, this seemed to make sense medically...so Americans have taken this nutritional advice. But if the statistics are a guide, our national low-fat, high-carbohydrate diet has been a miserable failure in the fight against obesity."

And finally, after criticism by the establishment for over two decades, some small studies are now supporting the Atkins formula—high protein, not high carbs—contribute to weight loss and better health.

A Duke University study found that patients on the Atkins Diet lost 31 pounds over six months, while a comparative group of subjects on the low-fat diet recommended by the American Heart Association lost only 20 pounds. In addition, only the patients on the Atkins diet enjoyed an increase in their levels of HDL—good cholesterol.

Critics point to the fact that the study was funded by the Atkins Center for Complementary Medicine, however, the findings were important enough for the National Institutes of Health to fund its own study through the University of Pennsylvania scheduled for completion in 2007.

What's The Answer?

Just as there seems to be no one single, simple cause for the rise in American obesity, so there may also be more than one solution. Should we diet? Should we work out? Should we have our stomachs stapled? Should we swallow pills and potions? Should we eat protein? Should we give up sugar? Should we eat off smaller plates? Should we stop watching TV? Should we...Should we...Should we? What should we do?

For now, prudence dictates that a compromise between the established recommendations for obesity management and some of the newer therapies may be the answer. A balance between the old and the new. With a large dose of common sense thrown in. And finally, an aggressive program of self-education, may provide the beginning of relief and the reversal of the obesity epidemic.

And by reading this book, you are already well along your own path to self education and new knowledge!

Chapter 3 How Fat Are You?

It may be that your pants are getting a little snug. Or you find yourself huffing and puffing when you go up a flight of stairs. Or your cholesterol levels are high. Or your doctor has told you to lose weight and get in shape. Whatever your motivator for starting a fat-reduction program, it's useful to take a measure of just where you fall on the obesity grid.

The Centers for Disease Control through the National Center for Chronic Disease Prevention and Health Promotion have selected three tests as measures of individual obesity.

But first, understand the definition of obesity, which according to the National Research Council is defined as an excessively high amount of body fat or adipose tissue in relation to lean body mass. The amount of body fat includes both the distribution of fat throughout the body— location, location, location—and the size of the adipose tissue deposits.

We now have three reliable measures of obesity: The BMI Test; the Waist Circumference Test; and the Waist-to-Hip Ratio Test. (However, total obesity or overall obesity is still more risky than body fat stored in specific areas of the body or the hip-to-waist ratio).

1. The Body Mass Index (BMI) Test

The BMI is based on your height and weight and is a helpful indicator of both obesity and underweight in adults.

There are many BMI calculators available on the Internet, to quickly and accurately calculate your BMI. But, for those who prefer a hand-held calculator, here is the formula to follow:

What's Your BMI?
BMI FORMULA: Your weight in pounds divided by your height in inches divided by your height in inches again and that figure multiplied by 703.

Example: A person weighing 210 pounds and 6 feet tall would have a BMI = 210 pounds divided by 72 inches divided by 72 inches multiplied by 703 = 28.5.

A healthy BMI for adults is between 18.5 and 24.9. BMI ranges are based on the effect body weight has on disease and death according to the World Health Organization. Research increasingly supports the fact that a high BMI is a predictor of risk factors and even death from cardiovascular disease, diabetes, certain forms of cancer, high blood pressure and osteoarthritis.

How do you rate?
Underweight	BMI less than 18.5
Overweight	BMI of 25.0 to 29.9
Obese	BMI of 30.0 or more

2. The Waist Circumference Test

This is a common measurement used to assess belly fat, or the abdominal fat content. Experts have found that this measure is an independent predictor of risk factors and health problems associated with obesity, when it is out of proportion to your total body fat.

What's Your Waist Circumference?
Stand up straight. Relax. Using a tape measure, measure the distance around the smallest area below your rib cage and just above your belly button.

How Do You Rate?
Men are at risk if waist circumference is greater than 40 inches.
Women are at risk if waist circumference is greater than 35 inches.

3. The Waist-To-Hip Ratio (WHR) Test

This is the ratio of your waist circumference to your hip circumference. The way to determine your waist-to-hip ratio is to measure your waist circumference and divide it by your hip circumference. Experts warn that for both men and women a waist-to-hip ratio of 1.0 or higher is considered "at risk" for obesity-linked health problems.

If your overall body fat and/or the results of these tests show you to be above the accepted medical limit, it is important for you to begin to take steps to bring your body to safer and healthier levels.

Chapter 4   Health Risks of Obesity

It almost seems unnecessary to list the many health risks associated with obesity from the most deadly and life threatening to those that restrict the overall quality of life. But, like all dangers, the dangers of obesity bear repeating until they have been finally and forever eliminated as risks.

Obesity As A Chronic Disease

In 1998, the National Heart, Lung, and Blood Institute (NHLBI) Obesity Education Initiative in cooperation with the National Institute of Diabetes & Digestive & Kidney Diseases (NIDDK) released the *Practical Guide on the Identification, Evaluation and Treatment of Obesity in Adults*. This publication demonstrated to the public and health care professionals alike that the government was committed to the management of obesity as a chronic disease and as a public health problem.

The Centers for Disease Control consider overweight and obesity to be chronic diseases of epidemic proportions and an independent risk factor for cardio vascular disease.

In addition, obesity and overweight aggravate risk factors already present such as an established history of coronary heart disease; atherosclerotic diseases; Type-2 diabetes; sleep apnea; hypertension; elevated LDL cholesterol; impaired fasting glucose; family history of premature CHD; and age.

Chapter 5   Fat-to-Fit-to-Fat Yo-Yo

Up until now these were the options opened to anyone who wanted to get control over their rising body fat levels. Here's what the experts have been saying are the current options for successful fat loss and weight management.

Adjust Your Diet For Weight Loss

The CDC recommends a conservative weight loss program of 1 pound per week achieved through reducing daily calories by 500 to 1,000 per day. They also recommend a diet of 1,000 to 1,200 calories per day for women and 1,200 to 1,600 calories per day for men.

Add Daily Exercise To Your Life

Physical inactivity is closely associated with the increase in obesity. The NHLBI guidelines recommend that physical activity be a part of weight-loss therapy and weight management, going on to state that adding regular activity to a calorie restricted diet program can accelerate weight loss and increase the overall amount of weight lost by 4-7 pounds. Even better news, is that people who integrate an exercise program as part of their overall weight loss plan have a much greater success rate at keeping weight off. The NHLBI guidelines suggest a moderate amount of physical activity at the beginning increasing to at least 30 minutes of more intense physical activity on most—and preferably all—days of the week.

Keep A Journal

The Centers for Disease Control recommend keeping a weekly food and activity journal or diary because record-keeping has been shown to be one of the most successful behavioral techniques for both weight loss, and post weight-loss maintenance. The journal should be reviewed weekly, with a health care professional, and should include records of diet, physical activity and behavior goals.

Get Educated

It isn't enough to just want to lose…you need to learn how to lose. Take some time each week to read the latest books or magazines or journals on nutrition and weight loss. Visit the many nutritional web sites. Go into the chat rooms. Listen. Learn. Lose.

Go For The First 10%

The initial goal of a good weight loss program goes for the first 10% of body weight. Just by achieving a loss of 10% of your body weight has demonstrated significant decrease in the development of diabetes, hypertension, and other obesity related diseases.

Drugs

Some, with guidance from their own health care professionals, may benefit from anti-obesity drugs. But anti-obesity drug therapy can be dangerous—even life threatening. Remember the dexfenfluramine and fenfluramine combo that was approved with such fanfare but was withdrawn when it was found that the drug was linked to potentially fatal complications. The NHLBI obesity guidelines recommend that overweight individuals with a BMI greater than or equal to 27 kg/m2 and "concomitant obesity-related risk factors or diseases" or obese people with a BMI greater than or equal to 30 kg/m2 and no concomitant disease be considered candidates for weight-loss drugs.

Surgery

This is an increasingly popular but still dangerous alternative therapy that has recently enjoyed a great deal of media attention. However, most experts agree, that much more study of the long term effects is needed before it can be widely recommended.

The Future Of Final Fat Loss Is NOW!

Research continues. Everything from new drugs, new herbal offerings, hormones, proteins, almost everything that can remotely fight the obesity battle is being researched and tested.

But it is only recently that a real breakthrough has been made which may hold the nutritional key to bring a relief and success to the millions of Americans who are trapped in even larger prisons of fat.

Part Two

The Calcium Part

Chapter 6   The Calcium Crisis

1994

In June 1994, The National Institutes of Health Consensus Panel on Optimal Calcium Intake first encouraged professionals in health and nutrition to work together to increase Americans' dietary calcium intake.

The recommendations and conclusions arrived at were based on data and research available at the time:

A large percentage of Americans fail to meet currently recommended guidelines for optimal calcium intake.

On the basis of the most current information available, at that time, optimal daily calcium intake from both, calcium from the diet, and from supplements was estimated as follows:

Infants Birth to 6 months	400 mg
Infants 6 to 12 months	600 mg
Young children 1 to five years	800 mg
Young children 6 to 10 years	800 mg to 1200 mg
Age 11 to 24	1200 mg to 1500 mg
Women 25 to 50	1000 mg
Pregnant or lactating women	1200 mg to 1500 mg
Post menopausal women on estrogen replacement therapy	1000 mg
Post menopausal women not on estrogen replacement therapy	1500 mg
Men 25 to 65	1000 mg
Men and women over 65	1500 mg

Note: New Guidelines in Reference Section.

Adequate vitamin D is essential for optimal calcium absorption. Dietary constituents, hormones, drugs, age, and genetic factors influence the amount of calcium required for optimal skeletal health.

Calcium intake, up to a total of 2000 mg/per day, appears to be safe in most individuals.

The preferred source of calcium is through calcium-rich foods such as dairy products. Calcium-fortified foods and calcium supplements are other means by which optimal calcium intake can be reached in those who cannot meet this need by ingesting conventional foods.

A unified public health strategy is needed to ensure optimal calcium intake in the American population

The research at that time into the effect of calcium on reducing preeclampsia was found to be insufficient but warranted further study. At this time it was also found that the preliminary research indicating that increased calcium may lower the risk for developing colon cancer was also insufficient. And finally, even though there were a number of studies that showed the relationship between blood pressure levels and calcium intake, it was hoped that more research would be forthcoming.

It was pointed out during this meeting that increasing calcium intake might interfere with the absorption of other nutrients or increase gastric acid secretion. However, these risks were found to be acceptable and a maximum of 2000 mg of calcium per day was settled on as a safe limit that would not produce adverse effects.

The final report from this meeting states, "Optimizing the calcium intake of Americans is of critical importance. Recent improvements in calcium intake have been reported for most age groups (phase I of the Third

National Health and Nutrition Examination Survey, 1988-1991—NHANES III). However contemporary 6-to 11-year old children showed a decrease in calcium intakes, as compared with those a decade earlier (NHANES II, 1976-1980). NHANES III also documents that a large percentage of Americans still fail to meet currently recommended guidelines for calcium intake. The impact of sub-optimal calcium intake on the health of Americans and the health care cost to the American public is a vital concern. It is thus appropriate that increasing calcium intake is a national health promotion and disease prevention objective in the *Healthy People 2000* agenda."

1999

Five years later, in June 1999 nearly 50 representatives from national health and nutrition organizations met in Washington, D.C. for a national Calcium Summit. This landmark meeting was hosted by the National Dairy Council and Milk Processors Education Program.

Why such a meeting? What caused the calcium crisis? What kept America in a calcium crisis? The answer, in part was offered during the keynote address delivered by an Under Secretary of the U.S. Department of Agriculture, who suggested that a dramatic decline in milk consumption, particularly among children and teens may account for part of the problem.

In fact, new educational initiatives from the Department of Health and Human Services and the National Institute of Child Health and Human Development had been developed to encourage children and teens to drink more milk, since studies were increasingly revealing that milk is one of the best sources of calcium and also, as a nutritional bonus, provides other nutrients, including vitamin D, which helps the body absorb calcium.

As a result of the Calcium Summit, leaders from 28 nutrition and health organizations signed on to a Calcium Coalition and dedicated themselves to "optimizing the calcium intake of Americans to help improve health and reduce chronic disease risk." And what were their recommendations?

- Raise the visibility of the country's calcium deficiency by educating targeted professionals.
- Repeatedly communicate consistent dietary calcium messages to consumers.
- Encourage increased distribution channels for high-calcium foods (food marts at gas stations, convenience stores, fast food chains, etc.).
- Publicize other developments, such as innovative milk packaging, to make milk more available and convenient.
- Make the Calcium Summit the starting point for a dialogue among leading health organizations.
- Implement "Mini-Calcium Summits" across the country.

In addition to the recommendations put forth, there were several exciting research reports discussed or presented.

Calcium & Dairy-Sourced Calcium: According to researchers at Creighton University, who addressed the Calcium Summit meeting, the calcium found in milk is an essential nutrient. Further a variety of studies show powerful health benefits from what scientists are now calling calcium—a super-nutrient. A calcium deficiency has been linked to osteoporosis, high blood pressure, colon cancer, kidney stones, obesity and even premenstrual syndrome.

Calcium & Hypertension: A spokesperson from Oregon Health Sciences University added that a review of studies showed that calcium can lower blood pressure, but that milk has an even stronger effect. The DASH study (Dietary Approaches to Stop Hypertension) linked a diet rich in low fat dairy, fruits and vegetables to lowered blood pressure in people with mild hypertension, by as much as some medications, and went on to suggest that if the DASH food plan were more universally adopted, the United States could see a 27 percent reduction in the incidence of stroke and a 15 percent reduction in the incidence of coronary disease.

Calcium & Colon Cancer: There's more. In a human clinical trial, at Columbia University, College of Physicians and Surgeons, preliminary results showed that low fat dairy products produced beneficial changes in the biomarkers for colon cancer. It was suggested that perhaps other factors in the dairy foods, such as vitamin D, may play a role in this encouraging and developing research.

Milk Matters Campaign: The National Institute of Child Health and Human Development launched a campaign called Milk Matters targeted at America's younger generation. Why? Because experts feel strongly that osteoporosis, the disease that has been until now associated with mature women, is a pediatric disease with geriatric consequences. That the careful attention to calcium, especially in dairy products, at an early age, could help avoid future health problems in maturity.

Reaffirmation of the DASH Diet: The DASH diet was reaffirmed, high in low fat dairy, fruits and vegetables resulting in a diet rich in calcium, potassium and magnesium was cited by both the American Heart Association and the National Heart, Lung, and Blood Institute as one method for preventing and treating high blood pressure.

The National Bone Health Campaign: The Office on Women's Health at the U.S. Department of Health and Human Services also introduced a new program, called the National Bone Health Campaign, targeted at teen age girls, who experts believe get less calcium from dairy than teenage boys. The effort was developed in an attempt to help prevent osteoporosis and reduce the 1.5 reported fractures attributed to osteoporosis and the billions of dollars in health costs related to the disease.

Obesity: Some of the earliest studies linking obesity to calcium intake levels were also reported. Preliminary research from scientists at Purdue University found that when women who consumed a diet containing less than 1900 calories per day also consumed at least 780 mg of calcium per day, they either lowered or maintained their body fat. Women, on the other hand, who consumed the same diet of less than 1900 calories per day, but who consumed less than 780 mg of calcium per day actually gained body fat.

2001

The National Institutes of Health, National Institute Of Child Health and Human Development in December 2001 issued a News Release stressing the importance of informing children about the dangers of low calcium intake." Only 13.5 percent of girls and 36.3 percent of boys age 12 to 19 in the United States get the recommended daily amount (RDA) of calcium, placing them at serious risk for osteoporosis and other bone diseases, according to statistics from the U.S. Department of Agriculture." The news release goes on to state, "Because nearly 90 percent of adult bone mass is established by the end of this age range, the nation's youth stand in the midst of a calcium crisis."

The seriousness of the issue was underscored by expert reports from the National Institute of Child Health and Human Development (NICHD), sponsor of the Milk Matters calcium education campaign who stated, "Osteoporosis is a pediatric disease... during these important bone growth periods, today's children and teens are certain to face a serious public health problem in the future."

The news release announced the expanded information base on the government website, targeted to children directly. Explaining that "previously, the NICHD developed educational materials that are used primarily by educators, nurses, and physicians to convey the importance of adequate calcium consumption among children and teens. Now, NICHD has expanded its Web site to give children and their parents more direct access to the information..."

The NICHD recommendations for calcium intake for children and teens are based on the "1994 National Institutes of Health (NIH) Consensus Development Conference on Optimal Calcium Intake, and on additional guidance from the 2000 NIH Consensus Development

Conference on Osteoporosis Prevention, Diagnosis and
Therapy."

And from The American Academy of Pediatrics,
"Recent studies and dietary recommendations have
emphasized the importance of adequate calcium nutrition in
children, especially those undergoing the rapid growth and
bone mineralization associated with pubertal development.
The current dietary intake of calcium by children and
adolescents is well below the recommended optimal levels.
The available data support recent recommendations for
calcium intakes of 1200 to 1500 mg/day beginning during
the preteen years and continuing throughout adolescence as
recommended by the National Institutes of Health
Consensus Conference and the National Academy of
Sciences."

2002

On January 17, 2002 experts gathered in
Washington D.C. to develop an action plan to address a
critical health concern facing children and adolescents:
calcium deficiency. According to a press release issued by
the National Dairy Council, "Government data indicates
that calcium intake remains dangerously low in the diets of
children and adolescents…" Speakers blamed the
combination of too much low nutrient foods and too little
consumption of nutrient-rich foods such as milk. "The
problem is particularly troubling for teens:
nearly nine out of 10 girls and seven out of 10 boys fail to
meet current calcium recommendations (1300 mg/per day
for ages 9 to 18)." The blame for the calcium deficiency
was in part directed to the easy availability of soft drinks in

schools and the fact that teenagers drink twice as much soda as milk, with potentially drastic health implications. The release goes on to report that "The American Academy of Orthopedic Surgeons (AAOS) was one of more than 40 organizations that supported the mission of Calcium Summit II to help America's youth make improved dietary choices to achieve optimal calcium intakes."

So the evidence is in. Calcium is important for everyone virtually from the youngest infant to the most senior, senior. And now comes the excitement from new breakthrough research into this most extraordinary super nutrient.

Chapter 7   New Calcium Science

Every year more and more studies report a wide variety of health benefits from calcium. Experts virtually all agree that every segment of the U.S. population can benefit from calcium in their diet—women, children, teenagers, men, unborn babies, and the elderly.

The Gale Encyclopedia of Alternative Medicine, the North American Menopause Society Expert Consensus Committee 2001 and others, cite research that points to calcium's growing role as a major contributor to health. Here's what the growing body of research is reporting:

Pregnancy
A study in the October 1999 issue of the *Journal of Obstetrics & Gynecology* found that pregnant women who do not get enough calcium in their diet can increase the bone mineral content of their fetus by about 15% by taking 1300 mg of calcium supplement per day during their second and third trimesters.

PMS
Researchers at the National Institute of Mental Health (NIMH) found that women who took 1200 mg of calcium per day reduced their overall PMS symptoms by more than 50%. The study also found that PMS mood swings were reduced by 45%, food cravings were reduced by 54% and bloating and water retention was reduced by 36%.

Stroke
Women in the Nurses' Health Study who took more than 400 mg of calcium daily were at the lowest risk for stroke.

Dental Health
Dental researchers at the State University of New York at Buffalo report that calcium supplementation may prevent periodontal disease since calcium helps build a strong jaw bone.

Colon Cancer
A brief article that was published in the *Journal of the American Dietetic Association* in 2001 from the *Lancet* reporting on a study conducted by the European Cancer Prevention Organization Study Group, which found that "fiber and calcium supplementation may prevent colorectal cancer relapse."

Prostate Cancer
One 2001 study conducted at Harvard Medical School found that those men who consumed the most calcium and dairy products had a greater risk of prostate cancer.

Osteoporosis
Calcium and vitamin D are both essential components of osteoporosis therapy with all anti-resorptive agents.

Colorectal Cancer
Based on the generally consistent animal and human data, a case can be made that high calcium intake provides some chemo protective properties against colorectal cancer. The data are not sufficient to support a general recommendation that women take calcium solely to prevent colorectal cancer. However, since women should consume at least a minimum amount of calcium required for skeletal health, they may receive an added colorectal cancer benefit.

Hypertension
Trials have demonstrated that calcium intake is associated with a beneficial effect of hypertension. However, the data are not sufficient to support a general recommendation that women take calcium solely to prevent or treat hypertension. Women may experience an added hypertension benefit from consuming the minimum amount of calcium required for skeletal health.

Obesity
Although limited data suggest a statistically strong, inverse correlation between the risk of obesity and dietary calcium intake, available studies indicate that calcium intake explains only a small portion of the variability in body weight in postmenopausal women. Nevertheless, as for the other non skeletal disorders addressed in this consensus opinion, ensuring an adequate calcium intake for skeletal purposes may confer small weight-control benefits as well.

So, as research progresses, the excitement mounts, particularly since there are now strong and compelling research indicators that point to calcium as the key to unlocking America's fat cells and restoring America's lean, fit, health.

Chapter 8

The Miracle of
The Super Nutrient Calcium

Calcium Sources

There are two major sources of calcium available. One is the calcium found in foods and the other is in calcium found in supplements. Dietary calcium, found in foods is the best source of calcium. However, experts agree that most Americans do not eat a diet sufficiently high in dietary calcium on a daily basis and so adding calcium supplements may provide the additional calcium required for good health.

So let's take a look at the various sources of calcium: dairy such as milk, cheese and yogurt; non-dairy such as vegetables, fish, fruit and more; and calcium supplements.

1. Calcium & Dairy Sources

One of the best, richest sources of calcium is dairy food. Milk, yogurt, cheese are among the calcium superstars—and the best of these are the ones that are reduced in fat. Today several brands of milk are reinforced with additional calcium and those would be excellent choices to add to your shopping cart.

Milk

The National Dairy Council offers this breakdown of the composition of milk:

Milk Proteins: Milk proteins are composed of 20 different amino acids, 8 of which are considered essential because our own bodies are incapable of manufacturing them.

Minerals: Four vital minerals are found in milk—calcium, phosphorous, magnesium and zinc.

Vitamins: A rich source of vitamins, milk contains the fat-soluble vitamins A and D, as well as several of the B vitamins, including thiamine, riboflavin, niacin and B12.

It's important to get to know your milk.

Whole Milk: Whole milk must contain at least 3.25 percent milk fat and 8.25 percent milk solids. Most milk sold in the United States is fortified with vitamin D. Vitamin D is critical to the absorption of calcium.

Low Fat Milk: Low fat milk contains anywhere from 0.5 to 2.0 percent milk fat. Low fat milk is also fortified with vitamin D. In addition, low fat milk has added vitamin A because removing fat from milk, also removes vitamin A. Removing some of the fat does not remove calcium from milk.

Skim Milk: This milk has less than 0.5 percent milk fat and is also fortified with vitamin D. In addition, low fat milk has added vitamin A because removing fat from milk, also removes vitamin A. Removing some of the fat does not remove calcium from milk.

Chocolate Milk: Chocolate milk is made by adding chocolate or cocoa and a sweetener to milk. Chocolate contains oxalic acid which is a calcium blocker. There is generally not enough chocolate in chocolate milk to significantly affect calcium absorption.

Evaporated Milk: This involves evaporating enough water from milk to reduce its volume by half. The resulting milk is homogenized, fortified with vitamin D, canned and heat sterilized. It contains at least 7.25 percent milk solids.

Evaporated Skim Milk: This involves the same process as for evaporated milk. Vitamins A and D are added. Skim milk contains up to 0.5 percent milk fat.

Sweetened Condensed Milk: This canned concentrate of whole or skim milk is sweetened. The same vitamins and milk fat content apply as for whole or skim milk.

Cultured Buttermilk: Buttermilk is the result of adding a bacterial culture to skim or low fat milk. Salt is often added for extra flavor.

Storing Milk Safely

Because fresh milk is perishable it must be refrigerated at 40°F or less. The same is true for dry skim milk that has been mixed with water to form a liquid milk, and the same for canned evaporated milks. Pour only what you need and return the rest to the fridge, keeping the carton tightly sealed to prevent the milk from absorbing other food flavors in the fridge.

Calcium Content In Milk

Type of Milk	Calcium in mg
Sweetened condensed whole milk (4 ounces)	434
Evaporated skim milk (4 ounces)	369
Evaporated whole milk (4 ounces)	329
Skim milk (8 ounces)	316
Low fat milk 1% (8 ounces)	300
Low fat milk 2% (8 ounces)	296
Whole milk (8 ounces)	290
Cultured buttermilk (8 ounces)	285
Chocolate milk, low fat 2% (8 ounces)	284
Chocolate milk, whole (8 ounces)	280
Eggnog (4 ounces)	165

Cheese

Not all cheese is created equal, at least from a calcium point of view. Here are the calcium values in some of the more common cheeses according to the USDA. Today certain brands of cottage cheese, which had been one of the poorest sources of calcium, have now been reinforced with additional calcium, and these calcium-enriched products are better nutritional selections.

Type of Cheese (1-ounce)	Calcium in mg
Parmesan	355
Romano	301
Gruyere	287
Swiss	272
Provolone	214
Monterey	211
Mozzarella (part skim)	207
Edam	207
Cheddar	204
Cottage Cheese	19
Muenster	203
Tilsit	198
Gouda	198
Colby	194
Brick	191
Roquefort	188
American processed	174

Yogurt

In the early 1900s, Dr. Metchnikoff, a Nobel prize-winning scientist and friend of Louis Pasteur, the other famous name in dairy products, conducted a series of experiments with sour milk, believing that sour milk contained important elements that enhanced health. When his experiments showed mice fed a form of sour milk lived longest, had the healthiest babies and the cleanest internal organs, Dr. Metchnikoff believed he had found one of the secrets, if not to the fountain of youth, then at least to the fountain of health and longer life. Soon, the folklore about the healing and longevity properties of this special sour milk spread, and today, contemporary scientists are rediscovering the health benefits of what we know as yogurt.

Today studies are under way to validate the earlier experiments and to show that yogurt with its active cultures is a powerful immune system enhancer, infection fighter and may even prove to be a nutritional tool fighting certain forms of cancer.

Lactose Intolerance

It is estimated that over 30 million Americans are lactose intolerant and over 10 million Americans suffer from a milk allergy.

Lactose intolerance is very common, worldwide. In fact, over eighty percent of non-whites are lactose intolerant. Why? Because the enzyme lactase is not present in the small intestine. Lactase is important because it breaks down lactose, the carbohydrate of milk sugar, into simpler sugar molecules that can be absorbed. Without this enzyme, milk and cheese and some other forms of dairy food can cause cramps, gas, and even lead to gastrointestinal infections and inflammatory bowel disorder.

Lactose may also be called, milk solids, milk powder, dry milk, or whey powder.

Milk Allergy
Milk allergy is a sensitivity to the proteins in milk such as casein, lactalubmin and lactoglobulin. Milk allergy reactions may include eczema, asthma, wheezing, mucous build-up, diarrhea, vomiting and reddish or black circles around the eyes and earlobes.

Lactose Content In Dairy Foods

Food	Grams of Lactose
Dry milk, nonfat, ¼ cup	15.6
Dry whole milk, ¼ cup	12.3
Skim milk, 8 ounces	11.9
Low fat milk, 2%, 8 ounces	11.7
Whole milk, 8 ounces	11.4
Goat milk, 8 ounces	10.9
Evaporated milk, skim, 1 ounce	3.6
Evaporated milk, whole, 1 ounce	3.2
Half & Half, 1 tablespoon	6
Heavy whipping cream, 1 tablespoon	4
Light whipping cream, 1 tablespoon	4
American processed cheese, 1 ounce	2.5
Feta cheese, 1 ounce	1.16
Parmesan, 1 ounce	.91
Mozzarella, part skim, 1 ounce	.78
Gouda, 1 ounce	.63
Swiss, 1 ounce	.59
Ricotta cheese, part skim, ½ cup	6.37
Ricotta, whole, ½ cup	3.77
Cottage cheese, low fat, 4 ounces	3.07
Cottage cheese, creamed, 4 ounces	3.03
Cream cheese, 1 ounce	.75
Ice milk, vanilla, 1 cup	10.0
Ice cream, vanilla, 1 cup	9.9
Yogurt, plain, skim, 4 ounces	8.7
Yogurt, plain, low fat, 4 ounces	8.0

2. Calcium & Non-Dairy Food Sources

While dairy still provides the richest source of calcium, other foods can be used as sources of dietary calcium and added to the daily food plan. Here are some approximate values for non-dairy calcium-rich foods. Note, many foods you will find on your grocery shelves are now enriched with calcium, so when shopping always try to purchase the food with the most nutritional calcium value.

Food	Calcium in mg
Canned sardines with bones, 3 ounces	340
Canned mackerel with bones, 3 ounces	260
Canned salmon with bones, 3 ounces	200
Salmon, cooked, 3 ounces	130
Canned shrimp, 3 ounces	95
Oysters, 3 ounces	80
Clams, 3 ounces	60
Cooked lobster, 3 ounces	55
1 egg, extra-large	30
Tofu, processed with calcium sulfate Or calcium chlorate, 4 ounces	400
Tempeh, 4 ounces	170
Soymilk, fortified, 1 cup	160
Tofu, 4 ounces	130
Black-eyed peas, cooked, 1 cup	210
Soybeans, cooked, 1 cup	200
Lima beans, cooked, 1 cup	160
White beans, cooked, 1 cup	160
Black beans, cooked, 1 cup	135
Chick peas, cooked, 1 cup	135
Great Northern beans, cooked, 1 cup	130
Pinto beans, cooked, 1 cup	130
Navy beans, cooked, 1 cup	120
Dried beans, cooked, 1 cup	90
Collard greens, cooked, 1 cup	350
Bok choy, cooked, 1 cup	230
Turnip greens, cooked, 1 cup	230

Okra, cooked, 1 cup	220
Kale, cooked, 1 cup	180
Broccoli, cooked, 1 cup	160
Mustard greens, cooked, 1 cup	160
Rutabaga, cooked, 1 cup	100
Brussels sprouts, cooked, 1 cup	55
Cabbage, cooked, 1 cup	50
Nori, ¼ cup	300
Hijiki, cooked, ¼ cup	150
Wakame, cooked, ¼ cup	130
Agar-agar, 2 tablespoons	120
Kombu kelp, cooked, ¼ cup	75
Dried figs, 5 medium	135
Kumquats, 6 medium	65
Orange, 1 medium	55
Dates, dried, pitted, ½ cup	50
Raisins, ½ cup	50
Sesame seeds, 1 ounce	280
Almonds (shelled), ½ cup	190
Soy nuts, dry roasted, ½ cup	185
Walnuts, ½ cup	140
Hazelnuts, ½ cup	140
Tahini (sesame seed paste), ¼ cup	135
Brazil nuts, shelled, ½ cup	130
Sunflower seeds, hulled, 2 ounces	65
Orange juice, fortified, 1 cup	300
Grapefruit juice, fortified, 1 cup	280
Rice milk, fortified, 1 cup	240
Mineral water, 1 liter	200

3. Calcium Supplements

Ideally, the best way to nourish your body with sufficient calcium is through food. With careful attention to your diet, you should be able to select foods that will help you to take in the required daily calcium for optimum health and nutrition.

However, that is not always possible, and calcium supplements may be used to fill in any nutritional gaps in your daily diet.

The key, when selecting calcium supplements is to look for the "elemental calcium" on the ingredients label because not all calcium supplements contain the same amount of calcium. Why? Because there are different types of calcium, and each type contains different amounts of elemental calcium.

Comparison of Percentages of Elemental Calcium in Supplements

Type of Calcium	% of Calcium
Calcium carbonate	40
Calcium chloride	36
Calcium phosphate	30
Oyster shell	28
Calcium citrate	21
Calcium lactate	13
Calcium gluconate	9

Absorbability of Calcium Supplements

In order to test the absorbability of your calcium supplement, drop it into a glass of vinegar. It should completely dissolve in 30 minutes. If it doesn't it isn't sufficiently absorbable and you should consider switching to a supplement that will completely dissolve in 30 minutes in the vinegar test.

Calcium Supplement Usage Tips

Calcium supplements are called supplements, because they supplement the dietary intake of calcium, they should not be considered substitutes for good calcium nutrition.

Do not take more than 500 mg calcium supplements at one time, since large doses are not as readily absorbed as smaller doses taken several times a day.

Calcium is best absorbed when taken with food or with a glass of skim milk.

Calcium is less efficiently absorbed if taken too close to a high fiber food or meal.

Calcium is less efficiently absorbed if taken too closely to a high fat food or meal.

Calcium is less efficiently absorbed if taken too closely to any iron supplements you may be taking.

Calcium and iron should be taken at different intervals so as not to interfere with each other's absorption rates and abilities.

What Calcium Supplements To Take

There are many good calcium supplements available in your local pharmacy, health food store and grocery store. Look for reputable brands. And always check with your own health care professional to make sure your selection meets with their approval.

Supporting Nutrients

Nutrition doesn't occur in a vacuum. Calcium is part of a total nutritional symphony that enhances good health and longevity. Calcium needs nutritional support from other nutrients—vitamins and minerals to be efficiently absorbed into the body.

Vitamin D

Vitamin D is readily available by exposing your skin to 15 or 20 minutes of sunshine daily. This is generally enough to create 400 IU of Vitamin D the amount required for normal body function. Here is a double bonus—take a walk for exercise and at the same time, stock up on your vitamin D requirement.

Excessive use of sunscreen, northern climates with long, sunless winters, and being housebound, aging, and windowpanes that block natural sunlight are some of the factors that create a risk for vitamin D deficiency.

Additional dietary sources of vitamin D include milk, herring, mackerel, tuna, canned salmon, canned sardines, shrimp, eggs, and fortified cereals.

Phosphorous

Scientists believe that the ideal ratio between calcium and phosphorous in the body is 1:1 since phosphorous is an important mineral in bone health and calcium metabolism. The danger, however, seems to be not from too much calcium in the diet affecting the ratio, but from too much phosphorous.

Magnesium

Magnesium can be called one of the "key" bone minerals along with calcium and phosphorous.

Many Americans are deficient in magnesium. Enjoying a balanced diet supplemented with a good multivitamin offers protection against magnesium deficiency.

Good dietary sources of magnesium include tofu, pumpkin seeds, nuts, wheat germ, whole-wheat flour, legumes, fish and dried apricots.

Nutritional Support

Generally, a balanced diet and a good multivitamin daily will help to offset any deficiencies. However, it is always recommended that you check with your own healthcare professional to help you create a personalized, nutritional program that fits your own individual requirements and takes into account your own individual nutritional deficiencies.

Calcium Inhibitors

The calcium landscape is littered with nutritional landmines that can reduce the absorption of the daily calcium you ingest whether from dietary sources or through supplements. Some of these can increase the excretion rate of calcium through urine, robbing you of vital milligrams of absorbable calcium and negatively affecting your positive calcium balance. By recognizing these "calcium robbers" you can be on guard in your own daily diet—reducing them and increasing your calcium for optimum benefit and health.

Salt

Americans take in far too much salt every day. Salt is hidden in almost every single food we eat and many of us are guilty of sprinkling extra salt on all our meals from breakfast to dinner.

It is estimated that just 1 teaspoon of salt a day can cause a 1.5% decrease in bone mass per year, through increased calcium excretion through urine.

Many experts recommend no more than 2400 mg of salt per day—about one teaspoonful. The Sarah W. Stedman Center for Nutritional Studies at Duke University Medical Center recommends no more than 3,300 mg of salt daily.

Have a salt craving? Can't give it up? Salt is an acquired taste and can be modified. If you reduce your daily salt intake your taste buds will adjust to the reduction and your salt cravings will diminish after six weeks.

Researchers at Cornell University may have found a link between calcium and salt. Their early findings show that calcium deficiencies may trigger high blood pressure in people who are extra-sensitive to the blood-pressure-increasing effects of salt.

This link is confirmed by findings at the Mayo Clinic which reports that keeping your total salt intake to 1 teaspoon per day—and that includes all those hidden sources of dietary salt—may also help lower blood pressure.

Further along the same line of research, Arizona State University findings show that increasing calcium intake daily may lower blood pressure—if sodium reduction has no effect on blood pressure levels.

And finally, an encouraging study from Wayne State University in Detroit showed that men on a high-sodium diet were still able to lower their blood pressure by taking additional calcium.

On the international front, a study from New Zealand found that women taking the same amount of calcium every day had very different calcium results. Those on a high salt diet lost 30 percent more calcium than those on a low salt diet.

Even though many of these studies focused on calcium supplements, research at Cornell's Hypertension Research Center showed that increasing the amount of milk consumed daily may have a small effect on mild hypertension in the 90 to 104 range.

And finally, the National Heart, Lung, and Blood Institute confirmed the milk and high blood pressure link in a study that showed non-milk drinking men were twice as likely to have high blood pressure as those who drank a quart of milk a day.

Tips To Reduce Your Daily Salt Intake
- Get rid of the salt shaker on the table.
- Look for and buy low sodium canned foods.
- Taste your food before adding salt.
- Experiment with salt free seasoning, herbs and spices.
- Become a salt detective when reading labels. Salt by any other name is still salt: monosodium glutamate (MSG), Disodium phosphate, sodium bicarbonate (baking soda), sodium aluminum sulfate (baking powder), sodium benzoate.

Watch Your Intake of Salt-Loaded Foods

Sauerkraut	Dill pickles	Chicken broth
Soy sauce	Ham	Olives
Pretzels	Salami	Franks
Luncheon meat	Cheese spread	Caviar
Some mineral waters		

Caffeine

Although recent studies have confirmed that moderate coffee drinking does not have a negative effect on calcium, drinking more than 3 cups of coffee per day can drain vital calcium stores.

Several studies show that up to 31 percent of post menopausal women with significant bone loss drink four or more cups of coffee per day.

Coffee is not the only caffeine culprit. Tea and sodas also contain often high levels of caffeine.

Tips For Reducing Caffeine Levels

- Reduce the number of cups of coffee, tea, or sodas, per day.
- Switch to decaffeinated beverages.
- Add more water to your diet.
- Add skim milk as a beverage.

How Much Caffeine Are You Really Getting Daily?

Beverage	Caffeine in mg
Coffee, regular drip, 1 cup	130 approx.
Coffee, instant, 1 cup	60 approx.
Coffee, decaffeinated, ground, 1 cup	5 approx.
Coffee, decaffeinated, instant, 1 cup	2 approx.
Tea, 1 cup, 1 minute brewing time	20 approx.
Tea, 1 cup, 5 minutes brewing time	40 approx.
Instant, 1 cup	20 approx.
Iced, one can (12 ounces)	30 approx.
Milk chocolate mix, 1 ounce	10 approx.
Dr. Pepper (12-ounce can)	60 approx.
Mountain Dew	50 approx.
Regular cola (12-ounce can)	40 approx.
Diet cola (12-ounce can)	30 approx.

Alcohol

Here, as in so many things in nutritional health, the key is in moderation. There is evidence that moderate amounts of alcohol—particularly in red wine—may have a positive effect on cardiovascular health. And a study from Pittsburgh University found that 3 to 6 alcoholic drinks per week may raise estrogen levels in postmenopausal women and help conserve calcium stores in bones.

However, anything more than moderate drinking has a devastatingly opposite effect. Some research showed that excessive amounts of alcohol pull calcium directly from bones. And a Harvard study found that regularly drinking a substantial number of alcoholic beverages increased the likelihood of breaking both a hip and an arm. Researchers believe that alcohol may affect the delicate hormonal balance necessary to absorb and utilize calcium. Alcohol may also stimulate the increased production of urine, flushing out calcium before it can be utilized.

Nicotine
One of the single biggest causes of death in the United States is smoking—killing over 300,000 people per year.

Smoking has also been cited as the leading cause of stroke. Smokers are eleven times more likely to have a stroke, than nonsmokers. This is especially true for smokers under the age of 65. By quitting smoking, the risk of stroke is cut to that of a nonsmoker after five years for men, and just two years for women.

Smoking is especially devastating to calcium stores. Some studies show that smoking may damage the body's estrogen production ability, increasing the probability of thinning bones. It is also suspected that smoking may also block the calcium ingested from being absorbed.

The Osteoporosis Center at the Hospital for Special Surgery in New York found that smokers have twice as much chance of getting back fractures as nonsmokers—further evidence of the negative smoking and calcium-blocking relationship.

Excessive Protein

According Duke University Medical Center, "swift bone loss results from excessive protein intake. One study showed that women whose average daily protein intake was 65 grams, or about three hamburgers per day, excreted an extra 26 milligrams of calcium per day in their urine. Over one year, such calcium loss will probably result in a decrease in bone mass of 1 percent.

How much protein is enough? The Stedman Center, reports, "The National Academy of Sciences recommends that women eat 50 grams of protein daily, men 63 grams. The U.S. Department of Agriculture says that adults can ingest sufficient protein by eating two or three servings a day of 2.5 to three ounces each of protein-rich foods."

Excessive Fiber

While experts agree that Americans need to eat a high fiber diet—higher than is currently the norm for a large number of Americans, scientists believe that excessive amounts of fiber may have a negative effect on calcium absorption. According to the Stedman Center for Nutritional Studies at Duke University Medical Center more than 30 grams of fiber per day may contribute to bone loss and is not recommended for anyone at risk for osteoporosis.

Oxalates & Phytates

Oxalic acid, found in certain foods can hold the calcium in the intestine, not releasing it to the rest of the body.

Foods containing calcium-blocking oxalates include: asparagus, beets, chives, cocoa, dandelion greens, green beans, parsley, peanuts, rhubarb, sorrel, spinach, summer squash, Swiss chard, and tea.

Some nutritionists recommend adding a little vinegar or lemon juice to these foods, as the acid in the vinegar or lemon juice may help to release the calcium making more of it available and easier to absorb.

There are some greens that contain calcium, but are relatively low in oxalic acid. These include, endive, kale and turnip greens.

Phytates are phosphorous compounds found in bran or oatmeal and in legumes. These also bind with dietary calcium in the intestine.

A good rule of thumb, is to separate foods higher in calcium-binding properties from high-calcium foods and supplements to prevent excessive non-absorption.

Part Three

The Diet Part

Chapter 9   The Breakthrough Research

The research into the calcium-fat connection began over 10 years ago. Studies were independently going on in a variety of Universities including Harvard.

Early hints of the calcium-fat connection and the role calcium might play in the future well being, health, and slenderness of America came to light in the mid-1990s. A study released by the Department of Nutrition, University of Tennessee entitled, *The effects of calcium channel blockade on agouti-induced obesity*, concluded that "…agouti regulates FAS, fat storage, and possibly thermogenesis…and that Ca2+ channel blockade may partially attenuate agouti-induced obesity."

But the real excitement began in the year 2000 and is continuing and increasing as of this writing.

Studies at the University of Tennessee began to show that getting calcium through at least three 8-ounce glasses of milk daily could turn up the body's own fat-burning mechanism. Reports were coming in of researchers who had applied calcium-related fat-loss data found in laboratory mice to the American population by analyzing the National Health and Nutrition Examination Survey (NHANES III) data set and extrapolating from it the fact that body fat was lower in people who consumed more dairy products. And following up with a second study that found that a diet high in low fat dairy products may cause fat cells to produce less fat and begin a more efficient breakdown of already stored fat, resulting in lower overall body fat. The researchers described the results as "significant."

Other Universities contributed to the growing database. Purdue University found that women who consumed at least 780 mg of calcium every day, either lost body weight, or had less of an increase in their body weight over a two-year period, compared to a group of women who got less calcium.

In August of the same year, 2000, the journal, *Physiol Genomics* 2000 (Aug 9;3(2):75-82) published a further University of Tennessee study, *Role of intracellular calcium in human adipocyte differentiation,* which concluded that calcium indeed played a role in cellular fat regulation.

By November 2000 in an article in the *Journal of the American College of Nutrition* (Nov-Dec;19(6): 754-60) an article submitted by researchers at Purdue University, *Dairy calcium is related to changes in body composition during two-year exercise intervention in young women,* found that, "…subjects with a high calcium intake, corrected by total energy intake, and lower vitamin A intake gained less weight and body fat over two years in this randomized exercise intervention trial."

In February 2001 The University of Tennessee published further findings in the *FASEB Journal* 2001 (Feb;15(2):291-3. The article entitled, *Effects of dietary calcium on adipocyte lipid metabolism and body weight regulation in energy-restricted aP2-agouti transgenic mice,* reported that, "…increasing dietary calcium…will suppress adipocyte thereby facilitating weight loss…" Again, researchers stressed the calorie-restricted diet that was a component of the findings.

Spring found an article in the *International Journal of Obesity and Related Metabolic Disorders* (Vol.25). The role of dietary calcium and other nutrients in moderating body fat in preschool children was designed to assess preschool children's food consumption (24-60 months) and relate these findings to body composition at 70+/-2 months. The conclusions drawn were as follows: "Higher longitudinal intakes of calcium, monounsaturated fat, and servings of dairy products were associated with lower body fat."

And in June 2001 in a meeting researchers from the University of Tennessee reported that, "...clinical data demonstrating that increasing dietary calcium results in significant reductions in adipose tissue mass in obese humans as by NHANES III data demonstrating a profound reduction in the odds of being obese associated with increasing dietary calcium intake. Notably, dairy sources of calcium exert a significantly greater anti-obesity effect than supplemental sources in each of these studies, indicating an important role for dairy products in the control of obesity."

By late summer the International community had joined the calcium research excitement. The Department of Clinical Medicine, University "La Sapienza" in Rome published their study, *Intracellular energy signals and dietary calcium: a milky way to the physiological control of hyperphagia and obesity?*

In October 2001 at the American College of Nutrition annual symposium presenters from the University of Utah shared their findings which showed that calcium from milk group foods may help children maintain a healthy body fat percentage during the critical years of body fat development.

And a further article, October 2001 in the *Journal of the American College of Nutrition* (Oct;20(5 Suppl):428S-

435S;discussion 440S-442S) entitled, *Calcium modulation of hypertension and obesity: mechanisms and implications*, drew the following conclusion, "Indeed, laboratory, clinical and population data all indicate a significant anti-obesity effect of dietary calcium, although large-scale prospective clinical trials have not yet been conducted to definitively demonstrate the scope of this effect. Thus available evidence indicates that increasing dietary calcium intakes may result in reductions of fat mass as well as blood pressure."

On February 6, 2002 the National Institute of Child Health & Nutrition (NICHD) began a two-year study titled: *Supplemental Calcium In Overweight People.*

Calcium and obesity research had now attracted the attention of federal agencies. The NICHD stated "This study will examine the health effects of calcium supplements in overweight adults. Overweight adults often eat a diet low in calcium. Some studies have found low calcium intake in people who have some of the medical problems often seen in overweight adults. This study will see if extra calcium improves the health of overweight adults."

In offering further study details, the NICHD added: "An estimated 97 million people in the United States are overweight or obese, and therefore have an increased risk for a number of other obesity-related co-morbid conditions (such as hypertension, dyslipidemia, and Type 2 Diabetes) as well as for all-cause mortality. The total cost attributable to obesity amounted to $99.2 billion in the US in 1995 and this figure, like the prevalence of increased body mass, is rising at an alarming rate. At the same time calcium intake in the US adult population is far below the RDA (recommended daily allowance) and much below the daily optimal calcium intake recommended by the 1994 NIH consensus conference. An analysis of the NHANES III database suggests a strong inverse association between relative risk of obesity and calcium intake. Further, both prospective studies in animal models, and retrospective analysis of human studies suggest calcium supplementation may play a role in minimizing yearly weight gain, and may possibly induce small weight losses."

A month later, in March 2002 the *British Journal of Nutrition* (Mar; 87(3): 239-45) published a study from the Institute of Biomedicine, Pharmacology, University of Helsinki, Finland which focused on the reduction of LDL-cholesterol levels with the increase of calcium.

That spring of 2002, the *Journal of the American Medical Association* (*JAMA* 2002; 287: 2081-2089) reported a study undertaken by Harvard University, funded by the National Institutes of Health and co-sponsored by the National Heart, Lung and Blood Institute. The study, entitled *Dairy Consumption, Obesity and the Insulin Resistance Syndrome in Young Adults: The CARDIA Study,* found that participants who consumed the most dairy products had a 71 percent lower incidence of IRS (Insulin Resistance Syndrome) than those who consumed the fewest dairy products. Researchers believe that the calcium, potassium, magnesium and other nutrients found in milk may provide protection against diabetes and possibly heart disease, both risk factors linked to obesity.

By April 2002 two separate articles in the *Journal of the American College of Nutrition* again stressed the inverse relationship between calcium and fat loss. The University of Tennessee article, *Regulation of adiposity and obesity risk by dietary calcium: mechanisms and implications*, reported that "…high calcium diets markedly inhibit lipogenesis, accelerate lipolysis, increase thermogenesis and suppress fat accretion and weight gain in animals maintained at identical caloric intakes. Further, low calcium diets impede body fat loss, while high calcium diets markedly accelerate fat loss…" The study went on to report, "Notably, dairy sources of calcium exert a significantly greater anti-obesity effect than supplemental sources in each of these studies, possibly due to the effects of other bioactive compounds…indicating an important role for dairy products in the control of obesity."

The second article, that April in the *Journal of the American College of Nutrition* (Apr;21(2):152S-155S) came from Creighton University in Omaha, Nebraska. It stated in part that, "Data from six observational studies and three controlled trials…have been reanalyzed to evaluate the effect of calcium intake on body weight and body fat. Analysis reveals a consistent effect of higher calcium intakes, expressed as lower body fat and/or body weight, and reduced weight gain at midlife, and body fat accumulation during childhood."

And then, "Taken together these data suggest that increasing calcium intake by the equivalent of 2 dairy servings per day could reduce the risk of overweight substantially, perhaps by as much as 70 percent."

We now come to January 2003. And again, Creighton University research published in the *Journal of Nutrition* (Jan; 133(1): 268S-270S, *Normalizing calcium intake: projected population effects for body weight*, concludes, "Although calcium intake explains only a small fraction of the variability in weight or weight gain, shifting the mean of the distributions downward by increasing calcium intake can be estimated to reduce the prevalence of overweight and obesity by perhaps as much as 60-80%.

And our research for this book ends with a strong call to action by the National Institutes of Health, in February 2003 and published in the *American Journal of Clinical Nutrition* (Feb; 77(2): 281-7). The Unit on Growth and Obesity, Developmental Endocrinology Branch, National Institute of Child Health and Development, National Institutes of Health in Bethesda report, "Limited epidemiologic and experimental data support the possibility that dietary calcium intake plays a role in human body weight regulation."

And so the research continues. Fast. Furious. Life-saving for the millions of obese and overweight Americans with the super nutrient, calcium.

Chapter 10 About The Calcium Diet

What makes *The Calcium Diet* so special? Why should *The Calcium Diet* be an essential part of your health, fitness and weight loss program? How does *The Calcium Diet* work?

What makes *The Calcium Diet* so special?

The Calcium Diet is very special. It is based on the miracle mineral, calcium. And the new, exciting research that points to calcium as perhaps the weight-loss miracle America has been waiting and hoping for. The premise behind *The Calcium Diet* is supported by 10 years of research at some of America's most prestigious and forward-thinking universities that first made the exciting calcium-weight loss link. There are no "cooked up" testimonials here, just the testimony of scientists and researchers and the results from their studies that speak for themselves. There are no dangerous drugs here. *The Calcium Diet* is based on the miracle mineral calcium in both its low fat dairy form and/or non-dairy form, and/or in its supplement form and calcium as an important nutritional component of America's quest for health has the support of the National Institutes of Health, the Centers for Disease Control, The National Heart, Lung and Blood Institute, the American Heart Association, The American Diabetes Association and the list goes on and on. And now, the calcium-weight loss connection is currently the subject of a two-year government study by the NICHD.

But there is more—much more—to *The Calcium Diet* than weight-loss, although obesity, now recognized as a national epidemic is an important component of *The*

Calcium Diet. It is a lifestyle that can, according to even more research, reduce your risk for life-shortening diseases such as hypertension, stroke, osteoporosis, some forms of cancer, and more.

And with all this, with all these health benefits, *The Calcium Diet* is as close as your own fridge. *The Calcium Diet* is as close as your own local grocery store.

The Calcium Diet is based on the key nutrient, calcium. Enjoyed through low fat dairy and non-dairy food sources but also augmented with calcium supplements.

The Calcium Diet is fast. Fun. Inexpensive. Filled with variety. You can pour it. Shake it. Chew it. Mix it. You can flavor it. Cook with it. You can serve it up hot. Serve it up cold. You can enjoy it for breakfast. You can have it for lunch. You can serve it for dinner. You can indulge yourself with it for dessert. You can have it for snacks. You can have it at home. On the road. Eating out. *The Calcium Diet* is universal. And universally simple.

The Calcium Diet is as easy as a glass of skim milk. *The Calcium Diet* is as easy as a calcium supplement.

The Calcium Diet can be used as your only nutritional diet, improving your health and fighting obesity. Or, it can be incorporated into your favorite weight loss program with additional positive benefits derived from dietary calcium.

In fact, many weight loss programs, while low in calories may not provide you with the required amount of calcium for optimum health. So, SOLO or COMBO, *The Calcium Diet* can become part of your quest for health, longevity and freedom from the many risks associated with obesity.

How much can you lose?

Just in case you skipped the "How to benefit from this book" section, here it is again to reinforce the remarkable powers of this super nutrient based diet.

How much can you lose? How fast can you lose? How easy is it going to be? Here's a sneak preview.

Studies show that just by being on any diet that restricts calories, you can expect to lose about 8% of your body fat and up to 11% of your body weight. Now look what happens when you add calcium. You can increase your weight loss by 25% and your fat loss by a whopping 69%!

That means that whatever diet you are on—*The Calcium Diet* can help you improve your results by up to 25%! What does this mean in real numbers? O.K. ladies, if you weigh 160 pounds and you have a decrease of 25% in body weight—that's 40 pounds. Guess what? Now you weigh 120 pounds!

Men. If you weigh 220 pounds and you have a decrease of 25% in body weight—that's 55 pounds. Now you weigh 165 pounds! Do your own math on your own weight.

That means that *The Calcium Diet* alone or added to your favorite diet can help you lose up to 25% more weight than you would on any other calorie-restricted program just by itself and up to 69% more body fat than you would on any other program.

That's what makes *The Calcium Diet* so incredibly special and unique. Use it as your only diet. Add it to your favorite diet. Either way, you lose more fat and more weight than ever before. You can lose up to 25% more weight and up to 69% more fat with calcium.

What does that mean? Less body fat. A leaner shape. Lose up to 69% more fat from your tummy. From your waist. Lose up to 69% more fat from your thighs. From your back. Lose up to 69% more fat from your entire body and be rewarded with improved health, more energy, a reduced risk of fat-linked diseases, and the vanity factor of just plain looking and feeling better!

How fast? Studies now show that just by adding the equivalent calcium found in one glass of milk—300 mg you may begin to lose as much as six pounds! Add the calcium of 2 glasses of milk and that becomes 12 pounds! Keep it going!

Simple. Effective. Powerful. And the subject of dozens of new studies, reports, and experiments.

Just remember. Everyone is different. Unique. Special. Everyone loses at a different rate. And everyone has different health and nutritional issues. So remember, before beginning this, or any other health or weight modification program you should always check with your own health care professional.

Now, let's move on to the miracle of the super nutrient and *The Calcium Diet*.

How does the calcium part of *The Calcium Diet* work?
The calcium part of *The Calcium Diet* works in several different ways but remember, it is only effective through the addition of dietary calcium with a calorie restricted diet, and exercise:

1. It helps turn off the hormones that trigger fat storage.
2. It helps turn on the hormones that trigger fat burning.
3. It helps to shift your metabolism from fat storage mode to fat burning mode.
4. It fights your body's natural tendency, when faced with a reduced calorie diet to activate the "metabolic protection" mechanism which is the plateau effect, so frustrating to dieters.
5. It curbs hormonally stimulated cravings that can sabotage your weight loss program and efforts.

Let's Look At What The Mice Tell Us
Researchers believe that as dietary calcium intake increases, it acts at the cellular level to alter the body's energy metabolism so that more food is actually burned for energy, and less food is stored in fat cells as fat. In addition, researchers believed that hormones regulating calcium levels, both inside cells and outside cell walls, were key in whether or not fat was stored or burned, and that dietary calcium influenced the hormones.
The researchers at the University of Tennessee used mice that were genetically patterned to mimic human obesity patterns.

The mice were genetically engineered to express a gene called agouti in their fat cells. This gene is normally found in human fat cells, but not in mice. The agouti gene influences whether a fat cell burns energy-containing molecules or whether the fat cell convert the molecules to fat. In other words the agouti gene determines whether a fat cell become a "fat maker" or a "fat burner."

These mice were first "fattened up", on a low calcium, high fat/high sugar diet. All four groups showed an increase of 27% in body fat. Now these mice were put on a low-calorie diet for 6 weeks. Their meals contained 30% less energy or calories than they would normally eat. They ate at 70% of their normal rate. All groups of mice got the same low-calorie diet. All groups of mice got the same amount of exercise.

Obese Mice In Group 1

 Placed on a calorie-restricted diet.
 The equivalent low amount of calcium most
 Americans get about 500 mg per day
 Have an 8% decrease in body fat.
 Have an 11% decrease in body weight.

Obese Mice In Group 2

 Placed on a calorie-restricted diet PLUS a calcium
 supplement of calcium carbonate equal to a human
 dose of 1,600 mg of calcium.
 Have a 42% decrease in body fat.
 Have a 19% decrease in body weight.

Obese Mice In Group 3
>   Placed on a calorie-restricted diet PLUS medium-
>   dairy diet of nonfat dry milk to
>   substitute for an equal amount of dietary protein.
>   Have a 60% decrease in body fat.
>   Have a 25% decrease in body weight.

Obese Mice in Group 4
>   Placed on a calorie-restricted diet PLUS twice as
>   much high-dairy diet
>   Have a 69% reduction in body fat.

Additional Observations:
Low Calcium Mice: Core body temperature falls—measure
of basal metabolism
High Calcium Mice: Core body temperature rises—
measure of basal metabolism boosted to burn fat.

What about humans?

The mouse results were applied to humans through
an analysis of the National Health and Nutrition
Examination Study (NHANES III) data set. After
controlling for caloric-intake, exercise, physical activity
and other factors, the researchers determined that body fat
was significantly lowered in people who consumed more
dairy.

The Theory Behind the Calcium-Fat Loss Connection

Not yet certain exactly how calcium works its
miracle on our fat making and fat losing machinery,
investigators do know this. LOW calcium intake triggers a
RISE in a hormone called the parathyroid hormone from

four glands in the neck. This hormone stimulates bones to release some stored calcium into the bloodstream.

At the same time, the kidneys also deliver a hormone called calcitriol, an active form of vitamin D that is designed to increase your ability to absorb calcium. These two work together to regulate the absorption of calcium from the gut and its movement in and out of bones. But, the problem is, that both parathyroid and calcitriol also stimulate the production of fat and inhibit its breakdown. The result? One of the side effects of elevated levels of this parathyroid hormone and active vitamin D is an accumulation of calcium in fat cells.

Some researchers think—and they are still working hard in labs to definitely find out—that this calcium—somehow encourages fat cells to store fat and discourages the breakdown of fat. The result, according to this theory is more body fat. On the other hand, high levels of calcium, seem to suppress these fat making and fat storing hormones.

Calcium Can Help You Stop Gaining & Start Losing

Here are some excerpts from research that shows how exciting the calcium-fat loss connect really is:

Women who consumed at least 780 mg of calcium per day in their diets, either lost or had less of an increase in body weight over a two year period compared to a control group who got less calcium. Based on research from Purdue University.

A study of 800 young and middle-aged women found that those with the lowest calcium intake had the highest body fat levels. Based on research from Creighton University, Omaha NE.

A study of the health records of 575 women in mid-life, found that women with the highest calcium intakes didn't gain weight and those with the lowest calcium did. This study related to women's weight. Based on research from Creighton University, Omaha, NE.

A study of children between the ages of four and eight found that children who had diets supplemented with more calcium and protein from dairy foods did not gain as much body fat as children in the control group. Based on research from the University of Utah.

A study reported at the Experimental Biology Meeting showed that women who consumed less than 1900 calories per day and who had at least 780 mg of calcium per day, either lowered or maintained their body fat. BUT women who averaged less than 780 mg of calcium per day GAINED body fat. Also women who got calcium from dairy foods experienced greater weight loss benefits than those who used non-dairy sources or supplements. Based on research from Purdue University.

An analysis of the diets of thousands of participants in a major US food consumption study, found that women who consumed the most calcium, about 1300 mg per day were less likely to be obese, than women who consumed little daily calcium. Based on research from the University of Tennessee.

A diet low in calcium appears to stockpile fat in fat cells. A diet high in calcium appears to deplete fat in fat cells. A high calcium diet releases a hormone that sends "lose fat" signals to the body's fat cells. Based on research from the University of Tennessee.

More dietary calcium forces fat cells to burn more fat and not store more fat as part of a calorie-reduced diet. Based on research from the University of Tennessee.

Too little dietary calcium and too many calories lead to more fat storage and less fat burning. Based on research from the University of Tennessee.

In a recent study overweight people on a calorie-reduced diet, who took a calcium supplement lost 26% more body weight and 38% more body fat than people just on a calorie-reduced diet. Reported by *Prevention.com*.

"Low calcium diets impede body fat loss, while high calcium diets markedly accelerate fat loss in transgenic mice subjected to caloric restriction. These findings are further supported by clinical and epidemiological data demonstrating a profound reduction in the odds of being obese associated with increasing dietary calcium intake." Reported in the *Journal of the American College of Nutrition* 2002.

"...calcium may play a substantial contributing role in reducing the incidence of obesity..." Reported in the *Journal Nutrition 2003*.

The Dairy Component
First study 10 years ago found that African American men, who added two cups of yogurt daily to their diet, reduced their body fat by about 11 pounds. The main objective of this study was to find a link if any, between a diet rich in dairy and a reduction in hypertension. The bonus of this study was the first real clue of the importance of calcium and dairy calcium in obesity.

In an animal study, a diet highest in low fat dairy showed the most impressive results in controlling body weight and body fat. A similar, separate analysis of human data showed that higher dairy intake was associated with significantly lower risk of obesity. Reported in *The Federation of American Societies for Experimental Biology (FASEB) Journal.* 2000.

Women who consumed higher intakes of calcium from dairy foods experienced more significant losses in weight and body fat than those women who consumed calcium from non-dairy sources. Reported in the *Journal of Clinical Endocrinology and Metabolism* 2000.

Children who followed a diet rich in calcium and dairy foods had lower body fat than children with lower dairy calcium intakes. Reported in the *International Journal of Obesity* 2001.

African American women who had higher dairy calcium intakes had significantly lower BMIs (the amount of body fat in relation to your height and weight and one of the measures of overweight and obesity) than women with lower calcium intakes. Reported in the *Journal of American College of Nutrition.* 2002.

Among Puerto Rican children, obese girls consumed significantly less dietary calcium and fewer dairy foods than their non-obese counterparts. Reported in *The Journal of Nutrition.* 2000.

Men who consumed more calcium and more dairy foods had less body fat than men who consumed few dairy foods or calcium. Reported in *The Federation of American Societies for Experimental Biology (FASEB)* 2000.

Research from Purdue University found that women who consumed at least 780 mg of calcium per day in their diets either lost or had less of an increase in body weight over a two-year period compared to the control group who got less calcium. Reported in *The Journal of the American College of Nutrition.* 2000.

"Notably, dairy sources of calcium exert a significantly greater anti-obesity effect than supplemental sources in each of these studies, possibly due to the effects of other bioactive compounds...indicating an important role for dairy products in the control of obesity." Reported in *The Journal of the American College of Nutrition* 2002.

Journal of the American College of Nutrition April 2002. reports, "Data from six observational studies and three controlled trials...have been reanalyzed to evaluate the effect of calcium intake on body weight and body fat...Taken together these data suggest that increasing calcium intake by the equivalent of two dairy servings per day could reduce the risk of overweight substantially, perhaps by as much as 70 percent."

Calcium Can Help Your Health
The Calcium Diet does more than help you fight fat and your risk for obesity. *The Calcium Diet* can also help you improve your general health and future prospects for longevity and a higher quality of life.

Calcium TOO Low
The US Department of Agriculture's Nationwide Food Consumption Survey (1987 to 1988) found that the average dietary calcium intake in the United States was far below the suggested optimal calcium intake.

Calcium and Blood Pressure
Calcium may benefit heart health. Dietary Approaches to Stop Hypertension (DASH) study, published in the *New England Journal of Medicine* in 1997 found that a healthy diet that included two to three servings a day of low-fat, calcium-rich dairy foods reduced systolic blood pressure by 5.5 points and the diastolic blood pressure by 3 points more than the control group.

13-year study at the University of Southern California School of Medicine found that 1,300 mg of calcium per day reduced hypertension risk by 12 percent, while subjects under the age of 40 reduced their risk by 25 percent. These benefits are most pronounced in hypertensive subjects who are also salt sensitive, a characteristic of many African Americans.

The Calcium Diet

Calcium and Diabetes

A 10-year study from Harvard reported in the *Journal of the American Medical Association (JAMA)* found that participants who consumed the most dairy products had a 71 percent lower incidence of IRS—insulin resistance syndrome—a key risk factor for type 2 diabetes and heart disease.

Calcium and PMS

A study published in the *American Journal of Obstetrics and Gynecology* reported that of 497 women, half took 600 mg of calcium carbonate twice a day, while half took a placebo. The women who took the calcium experienced significantly fewer PMS symptoms than those who didn't. Why? Calcium is a hormone regulator. Researchers found that calcium had a major effect on irritability, cravings, mood swings and other symptoms of PMS.

The U.S. Department of Agriculture's Human Nutrition Research Center found that in a study of 10 women with PMS those five who took 1,300 mg of calcium per day were less irritable, weepy, and depressed and reported fewer back-aches, less cramping and bloating, than women who only took 600 mg of calcium per day.

Calcium and Cholesterol

A study at the Center for Human Nutrition at the University of Texas Southwestern Medical Center found that a diet high in calcium reduced the level of total cholesterol by as much as six percent and lowered LDL cholesterol (bad cholesterol) by 11 percent. There was no reported effect on HDL cholesterol (good cholesterol).

Calcium and Colon Cancer
Cornell Medical Center found calcium may protect against growths that become malignant in those prone to colorectal cancer.

Cancer and a Healthier Fetus
Rockefeller University researchers believe that calcium supplements can help ensure the health of the fetus. In a study of hypertensive women adequate calcium and vitamin D levels improved pregnancy outcomes.

Calcium and Prostrate Cancer
Harvard Medical School 2001 study of more than 20,000 men found those who consumed the most calcium and dairy products had a 30 percent greater risk of prostate cancer.

Obesity in America
According to the Surgeon General's 2001 "Call to Action to Prevent and Decrease Overweight and Obesity" in 1999 an estimated 61 percent of U.S. adults were overweight or obese and 13 percent of children and adolescents were overweight. Today there are nearly twice as many overweight children and almost three times as many overweight adolescents as in 1980.

American Institute of Cancer Research (AICR) found that increased weight also increases the risk of several kinds of cancer such as breast cancer, colon cancer, endometrial cancer, prostrate cancer, and kidney cancer. Researchers also found that regular physical activity plays a role in reducing the risk of cancer. American Institute for Cancer Research, October 11, 2001.

This is a call to action for your own personal health and well-being and that of those you love. Read. Learn. And make it your personal life mission to be slender, fit, and healthy for yourself and for those you love and who love you.

Chapter 11   Get Ready To Lose

Now you are ready to begin.

These first 21-days are your guide to *The Calcium Diet* you can follow for life—a thinner, healthier life for you and your family. Start with these 21 days, and then, develop your own calcium-rich food days using recipes rich in calcium and low in fat, selecting products enriched with calcium whenever possible, and learning to read labels to make the best possible calcium-rich and low fat choices.

THE RULES OF *THE CALCIUM DIET*

1. **EAT REAL FOOD**

2. **GET YOUR CALCIUM**

3. **EXERCISE DAILY**

1. **EAT REAL FOOD**
   For calcium to do its job it is important that you
   restrict your daily caloric intake.* This will not be
   difficult as I have based the program on the highly
   successful AM PM Food Clock I developed as part
   of my Skinny System. You will be eating high-fiber
   foods that block fat in the AM hours and switching
   to high-protein foods that burn fat in the PM hours.
   You will also be eating 7 meals a day.

2. **GET YOUR CALCIUM**
   Experts agree that it is important to keep your daily
   calcium intake between 1,000 and 1,300 mg per day
   by following the recommended daily allowance and
   not go over 2,000 mg of calcium per day.
   The Calcium Diet has been developed to maximize
   your food-derived calcium as much as possible with
   suggestions for calcium supplements when your
   food does not provide sufficient calcium.

3. **EXERCISE**
   Exercise at least 30-minutes daily for over-all
   health.

* Note: The CDC recommends a daily caloric intake of 1000 to
1200 calories for women and 1200 to 2000 calories for men. Many
of the calcium studies reported their findings based on a diet of
1900 or fewer calories daily.

Let's Look At A Typical Day On *The Calcium Diet*

The first thing you will notice is that there are 7 meals on *The Calcium Diet*. And these meals are divided into AM and PM meals. This is the key "Food Clock" that is the basis of my successful system. So, if you can tell time, you can lose fat, weight, and get fit, lean and healthier.

There are two what I call, "skinny" food groups.

1. The AM Food Group is made up of fiber and carbs and it blocks new fat from entering your fat cells. And this group had added calcium for extra fat fighting and for preventing the additional storage of fat in fat cells.

2. The PM Food Group is made up of protein and it burns and melts away the old fat already stored in your fat cells. And this group has added calcium for extra fat burn.

Skinny Food Group 1: AM Fat Blocker Foods

Fat blocker foods are high in fiber and complex carbohydrates and are eaten when your watch says AM. By eating fat blocking foods first thing in the morning and then throughout the early or AM part of the day, several things happen. You reduce the insulin spikes that lead to fat storage and obesity. You lay down a protective coating that reduces the absorption of any new fat you might ingest from entering fat cells, you begin to scrub out vascular lipids, and you slow down the rate at which your stomach empties, keeping your feeling of fullness and satisfaction lasting longer and preventing cravings and hunger pangs.

Fiber belongs to a branch of the carbohydrate family and is the part that is not digested, but passes right through our system and is excreted. Fiber has no calories. It doesn't add to the dietary calories we can store as fat.

Fiber doesn't break down in our digestive system, which means it can't be absorbed, so again, it can't add to our fat supply. Fiber helps us feel full, soothing our appetite triggering center so that we are better able to refrain from stuffing ourselves. Fiber blocks the absorption of dietary fat —and fat calories—in our intestines and moves it harmlessly through our digestive system and out as waste. Fiber, as new research is showing every day, can help lower our blood fat, reducing cholesterol levels and improving our vascular health. It has also been shown to have a positive effect in reducing our risk for certain cancers and diabetes. Finally, most of us don't get nearly enough fiber every day—only 10 to 15 grams—as opposed to the 25 to 30 grams nutritional experts believe is the ideal and healthy amount.

There are two types of fiber and both are needed to get skinny, fast.

Soluble Fiber: Think Gum

This is the fiber that dissolves in water, becoming sticky and gummy. It's the stickiness that attracts blood fat and cholesterol, pushing it out through your digestive system so it doesn't have a chance to be stored as fat. This is the fiber you think of when you think apples, oranges, broccoli, carrots, and potatoes. As it enters and passes through your system this soluble fiber helps lower cholesterol, reduces your risk for heart disease, improves blood sugar readings and in many cases helps lower blood pressure.

Insoluble Fiber: Think Sponge

This is the fiber you think of when you think of bran muffins, oat bran cereal, oatmeal or popcorn. When you eat this type of fiber and follow it with a big glass of water, the fiber swells up—like a sponge—absorbing the water. The now soft and spongy fiber pushes on and out through your intestines, carrying with it excess dietary fat. As it passes through you, studies show that it helps in your overall digestion, aids elimination, promotes regularity and helps keep bowels clean.

Best AM Fat Blocking Foods

Breads	Oatmeal	Dried Fruit	Beans
Waffles	Oatmeal cookies	Grapefruit	Pasta
Pancakes	Raisins	Peas	White Rice
Apples	Tortillas	Cereal	Brown Rice
Oranges	Bran cereals	Potatoes	Pineapple
Pears	Popcorn	Raspberries	Kiwi
Pretzel	Blueberries	Lentils	Waffles
Pancakes	Bagels	Corn	Grits

Skinny Food Group 2: PM Fat Burner Foods

Fat burner foods are foods high in protein, a thermic element that actually burns or melts fat by raising the body's metabolic rate. By eating thermic foods—foods that produce heat—hot calorie foods—you can burn off 15 percent of your daily calories just in the caloric energy you use to eat, digest and most importantly, process thermic foods. Your metabolic rate increases when you eat these foods because your body has to work very hard to break down and absorb the nutrients in these foods. This produces more heat. More calories are burned off. Fewer calories are available to be stored as fat. This process is called the thermic effect of food. The best thermic foods are those high in protein. By enjoying these foods in the afternoon and evening—during the PM hours of the day—our body can burn fat, while we are more sedentary and even overnight while we sleep. Allowing our own metabolic process to become the ultimate fat fighting instrument.

But not all foods produce the same thermic burn. Not all foods have fat burning hot calories. The best foods are protein-rich foods.

We can increase our metabolic rate through a diet high in thermic foods. Yes, we can actually burn more calories WHILE WE EAT! Look at it this way. Our own body is our best fat burning machine. Just at rest, doing nothing more strenuous than keeping us breathing and blinking our body uses up to 60 percent of the calories we consume. Any amount of physical exercise we do uses up another 25 percent of our calories. That leaves 15 percent. Increase the thermic foods, and you increase the number of calories burned off and reduce your body fat.

Activity	% of Calories Burned Off
Resting metabolic rate	60%
Physical exercise	25%
THERMIC FOODS	15%

Best PM Fat Burning Foods

Lean red meat	Pork	Low fat yogurt
Chicken	Turkey	Eggs
Lamb	Fish	Skim milk
Tofu	Cheese	

Seven Meals Per Day

By eating frequently, you will be able to keep your body working to fight fat at a steady pace and you will keep a steady flow of calcium in your system at all times with its extra fat fighting metabolic power.

AM Meals

You will enjoy these AM meals daily. A pre-breakfast. A breakfast and a morning snack.

PM Meals

You will enjoy these PM meals daily. An afternoon snack. Dinner. A bedtime snack.

LUNCH AM or PM—The Choice Is Yours

Lunch is your choice. AM (fat blocking meal) or a PM (fat burning meal). AM is slower weight loss. PM is faster.

But first, take a look at the charts included here. This is a very real, and visual way for you to chart your progress in losing fat pounds and fat inches.

Tracking Your Weight Loss

Each time you lose a pound, cross it off this chart. And remember, before you begin, cross off all the pounds up to your starting weight.

350	349	348	347	346	345	344	343
342	341	340	339	338	337	336	335
334	333	332	331	330	329	328	327
326	325	324	323	322	321	320	319
318	317	316	315	314	313	312	311
310	309	308	307	306	305	304	303
302	301	300	299	298	297	296	295
294	293	292	291	290	289	288	287
286	285	284	283	282	281	280	279
278	277	276	275	274	273	272	271
270	269	268	267	266	265	264	263
262	261	260	259	258	257	256	255
254	253	252	251	250	249	248	247
246	245	244	243	242	241	240	239
238	237	236	235	234	233	232	231
230	229	228	227	226	225	224	223
222	221	220	219	218	217	216	215
214	213	212	211	210	209	208	207
206	205	204	203	202	201	200	199
198	197	196	195	194	193	192	191
190	189	188	187	186	185	184	183
182	181	180	179	178	177	176	175
174	173	172	171	170	169	168	167
166	165	164	163	162	161	160	159
158	157	156	155	154	153	152	151
150	149	148	147	146	145	144	143
142	141	140	139	138	137	136	135
134	133	132	131	130	129	128	127
126	125	124	123	122	121	120	119
118	117	116	115	114	113	112	111
110	109	108	107	106	105	104	103
102	101	100	99	98	97	96	95

Tracking Your Inches Lost

Take a look at the standard size charts below and then track the number of inches to your goal.

MISSES Standard Size Chart

Petite

Size	2	
Bust	32 ½	
Waist	24	
Hips	35	

Small

Size	4	6
Bust	33 ½	34 ½
Waist	25	26
Hips	36	37

Medium

Size	8	10
Bust	35 ½	36 ½
Waist	27	28
Hips	38	39

Large

Size	12	14
Bust	38	39 ½
Waist	29 ½	31
Hips	40 ½	42

Extra Large

Size	XL	
Bust	41	
Waist	32 ½	
Hips	43 ½	

PETITE Standard Size Chart (5'4" and under)
P/XS

Size	2P	
Bust	32	
Waist	23 ½	
Hips	34	

P/S

Size	4P	6P
Bust	33	34
Waist	24 ½	25 ½
Hips	35	36

P/M

Size	8P	10P
Bust	35	36
Waist	26 ½	27 ½
Hips	37	38

P/L

Size	12P	14P
Bust	37 ½	39
Waist	29	30 ½
Hips	49 ½	41

WOMEN'S Standard Size Chart

1X

Size	14	16
Bust	40	42
Waist	31	33
Hips	42	44

2X

Size	18	20
Bust	44	46
Waist	35	37
Hips	46	48

3X

Size	22	24
Bust	48	50
Waist	39 ½	42
Hips	50 ½	53

Commonly Asked Questions Before You Begin

Can I make substitutions?
For the first 21-days of *The Calcium Diet* it is recommended that you follow the program as written.

What if I'm lactose intolerant?
Check with your own health care professional for ways of dealing with your lactose intolerance.

What if I'm allergic to something in the meal plan?
By all means check with your own health care professional and replace the food with a similar value calcium-rich selection from the food lists available at the back of the book.

I'm on another diet program can I still follow The Calcium Diet?
The Calcium Diet works SOLO as the only diet plan you may need and it also works in COMBO with other diet plans that may not be as rich in calcium. Check with your own health care professional to make sure that you are incorporating the principles of *The Calcium Diet* into whatever food plan you are on.

I'm taking medications can I still be on The Calcium Diet?
Study after study, as you have read in this book, promotes calcium as a mineral with many health benefits, including certain forms of cancer, heart disease, hypertension, diabetes and more. Again, always check with

your own health care professional before beginning any weight or health modification program.

I still don't get the AM PM thing?

It's very simple, when your watch shows AM, you'll enjoy foods that are higher in fiber and complex carbs and calcium which help to block fat. When your watch switches to PM you'll enjoy foods that are higher in thermic protein and calcium, which help to burn the fat you've already got. This is a particularly good way for women to eat, benefiting from the high protein of a thermic diet, but still able to enjoy the health benefits and real dietary satisfaction of a complex carb.

It seems like a lot of food. Do I have to eat everything?

One of the reasons that you may not be losing, is that you simply aren't eating enough. You should eat every meal, however, if you are really feeling full, then you can eat smaller portions. The idea is not to skip any meals so that your body doesn't go into "starvation mode" and to keep your blood sugar levels from spiking. But you should ask your own doctor about the validity of eating often on your own body's metabolism.

Can my family also be on The Calcium Diet?

Adding calcium both from low fat dairy foods and calcium supplements has been shown to benefit everyone from children to grandparents. But again, you are urged to see your own health care professional to make sure that *The Calcium Diet* is right for your family and to make sure the recommended daily allowances are tailored for each member of your family according to their age and sex.

How quickly will I lose? How much will I lose?

Everyone is different. Be patient. Follow the basic principles and you will be rewarded with better health and a more slender body.

What about exercise?

Exercise is important. It is recommended that you get at least 30 minutes, but better, 60 minutes of exercise daily. This is a regimen that you could do as a family for better family health.

What's the Personal Journal?

It is important to track your progress and focus for a few minutes every day on new behaviors that will help you lose successfully and keep slim for a long time to come. The Personal Journal in *The Calcium Diet* gives you reminders to track your own progress and help with getting and staying skinny and fit.

What about the recipes?

Good question. You'll notice that each category of recipes is clearly marked AM or PM to help you in determining when to eat what. Once you get the hang of it, you'll find it is simple and a way of eating you can incorporate easily into your life.

Can I switch meals?

You may swap like-meals: Breakfasts on one day with breakfasts on another; Dinners on one day with dinners on another; Morning Snacks on one day with Morning Snacks on another and so on.

Chapter 12   21 Days of the Calcium Diet

Week 1-Day 1

Pre-Breakfast
One orange, or apple, or pear or 1 cup of berries.

Breakfast
One waffle with 1 tablespoon syrup and 6 ounces nonfat fruit yogurt.

AM Snack
Pudding Cup: 6 ounces reduced fat pudding, any flavor and/or calcium supplement.

Lunch
One cup cream of tomato or cream of mushroom soup made with skim milk and served with one slice whole wheat bread, reduced fat mayo with lettuce and a slice of tomato.

PM Snack
Cheese Tray: One ounce reduced fat cheddar cheese and one ounce reduced fat Swiss cheese arranged with ½ cup fresh veggies.

Dinner
Grilled fish (6-ounces) served with 1 cup steamed broccoli topped with 2 tablespoons lowfat dressing and 1 grilled tomato topped with 1 teaspoon parmesan cheese.

Bedtime Snack
Frozen Treat: 1 cup reduced fat frozen yogurt and/or calcium supplement.

Exercise: Today begin your exercise program by writing down your exercise goals—30 to 60 minutes of exercise per day;

Personal Journal: Write in your starting weight, your measurements and the results of the three Calcium Diet tests.

Week 1-Day 2

Pre-Breakfast
One orange, or apple, or pear or 1 cup of berries.

Breakfast
One slice raisin bread with 1 teaspoon low fat cream cheese and 1 teaspoon all-fruit preserves.

AM Snack
Fruit & Sweets Snack: 1 medium apple and 2 fig cookies and/or calcium supplement.

Lunch
One small baked potato topped with ¼ cup nonfat plain yogurt mixed with ¼ cup salsa and 1 tablespoon chopped parsley or topped with ¼ cup nonfat plain yogurt mixed with 1 tablespoon reduced fat salad dressing.

PM Snack
Deli Snack: Two ounces of reduced fat cheddar or Swiss cheese & 1 slice nonfat deli ham or turkey.

Dinner
Six ounces broiled steak served with 1 cup mixed vegetables flavored with a squeeze of lemon juice and one salad made with 1 cup Romaine, 1 cup endive, 1 chopped tomato, 2 green onions, sliced thin, 1 tablespoon grated parmesan cheese and tossed with 2 tablespoons nonfat salad dressing.

Bedtime Snack
1 cup reduced fat frozen yogurt, any flavor and/or calcium supplement.

Exercise: Today get a check-up to make sure that you are in shape to begin an exercise program if you haven't exercised for a long time and are out of shape. When you get an O.K. from your own doctor, you are ready to begin.

Personal Journal: Make a note beside each meal that you ate today and any "extras".

Week 1-Day 3

Pre-Breakfast
One orange, or apple, or pear or 1 cup of berries.

Breakfast
One toasted English muffin spread with 1 tablespoon reduced fat cream cheese and 1 tablespoon all-fruit spread.

AM Snack
A Pudding Treat: ½ cup rice low fat chocolate or vanilla pudding and/or calcium supplement.

Lunch
One glass (6-ounces) tomato juice and one veggie wrap made with 1 corn tortilla, ½ cup shredded romaine lettuce, 1 chopped tomato, ½ cup shredded spinach, 2 green onions, chopped, 1 tablespoon chopped parsley and ¼ cup plain nonfat yogurt mixed with ¼ cup salsa.

PM Snack
Hot Chocolate Treat: 6 ounces chocolate skim milk heated and topped with 1 tablespoon reduced fat whipped topping.

Dinner
Grilled chicken (6-ounces) served with 1 cup steamed broccoli and 1 green salad made with 1 cup Romaine lettuce, 1 cup endive, 1 tomato, 2 green onions, 2 teaspoons chopped parsley, ½ cup cucumber, ½ cup radishes and drizzled with 2 tablespoons nonfat salad dressing.

Bedtime Snack
1 ounce reduced fat cheddar or swiss cheese and/or calcium supplement.

Exercise: Today is your prep day. Schedule time in your day for exercise. Make sure your exercise clothing is in good shape.

Personal Journal: Make notes today about your weight—remember to weigh yourself at the same time and congratulate yourself for being motivated to begin a program of weight management and better health.

Week 1-Day 4

Pre-Breakfast
One orange, or apple, or pear or 1 cup of berries.

Breakfast
One cup oatmeal made with skim milk and topped with 1 teaspoon brown sugar.

AM Snack
Berry Treat: 1 cup mixed berries topped with 2 tablespoons reduced fat fruit yogurt and/or calcium supplement.

Lunch
One hard-boiled egg served on a bed of green salad made with 1 cup Romaine lettuce, 1 cup endive, 2 green onions sliced, 1 tablespoon parsley, chopped and 2 tablespoons nonfat dressing.

PM Snack
Nutty Surprise: 6 ounces reduced fat frozen yogurt topped with 2 tablespoons chopped almonds or chopped peanuts.

Dinner
Baked ham (6-ounces) or two hamburger patties served with 1 cup steamed broccoli or mixed veggies sprinkled with 1 tablespoon parmesan cheese, 1 sliced tomato, 2 slices onion, topped with 2 tablespoons nonfat salad dressing

Bedtime Snack
1 ounce reduced fat cheddar or swiss cheese and/or calcium supplement.

Exercise: Post your exercise intentions on your dashboard, the fridge, on the side of your computer, your bathroom mirror—anywhere you can to be reminded about your good intentions to begin. Exercise motivation is your key, today.

Personal Journal: Keep up with your food entries and remember, every day you are getting slimmer and healthier.

Week 1-Day 5

Pre-Breakfast
One orange, or apple, or pear or 1 cup of berries.

Breakfast
One slice raisin bread with 1 teaspoon low fat cream cheese and 1 teaspoon all-fruit preserves.

AM Snack
Fruit & Sweets Snack: 1 medium apple and 2 fig cookies and/or calcium supplement.

Lunch
One small baked potato topped with ¼ cup nonfat plain yogurt mixed with ¼ cup salsa and 1 tablespoon chopped parsley or topped with ¼ cup nonfat plain yogurt mixed with 1 tablespoon reduced fat salad dressing or topped with melted cheddar cheese (2 ounces).

PM Snack
Cheese Snack: Two ounces of reduced fat cheddar or Swiss cheese.

Dinner
Six ounces broiled fish served with 1 cup mixed vegetables flavored with a squeeze of lemon juice and one salad made with 1 cup Romaine, 1 cup endive, 1 chopped tomato, 2 green onions, sliced thin, 1 tablespoon grated parmesan cheese and tossed with 2 tablespoons nonfat salad dressing.

Bedtime Snack
1 cup reduced fat frozen yogurt, any flavor and/or calcium supplement.

Exercise: Time to get started. The Centers for Disease Control recommend that you keep a pair of good walking shoes in your car so that you'll always be ready to start walking. Today, your goal is to walk for 10 minutes—twice between breakfast and bedtime.

Personal Journal: Record your weight today, the foods you ate and your growing positive feeling about yourself.

Week 1-Day 6

Pre-Breakfast
One orange, or apple, or pear or 1 cup of berries.

Breakfast
Six ounces nonfat fruit yogurt and ½ cup granola.

AM Snack
Popcorn Surprise: One cup air-popped popcorn tossed with 1 tablespoon grated parmesan cheese and/or calcium supplement.

Lunch
One cup cream of tomato soup made with skim milk and one green salad made with 1 cup Romaine lettuce, 1 cup endive, 2 green onions sliced, 1 tablespoon parsley, chopped tossed with 2 tablespoons nonfat dressing.

PM Snack
Turkey Roll: Turkey roll made with 2 slices deli turkey rolled in two large Romaine leaves.

Dinner
Grilled chicken, turkey, or 2 small pork chops (6 ounces) served with 1 cup green beans topped with 1 tablespoons sliced almonds and 1 cup steamed spinach tossed with 2 tablespoons nonfat dressing.

Bedtime Snack
Bedtime Shake made with 1 cup skim milk, crushed ice and a sprinkling of cinnamon or nutmeg and/or calcium supplement.

Exercise: Today increase your walking from 10 minutes twice a day to 15 minutes twice a day. Try to increase your pace, too. How about walking in the mall? Walking around the block? Walking to the store and back?

Personal Journal: Record your weight and your meals and remember you CAN reach your goals. You are not alone.

Week 1-Day 7
Pre-Breakfast
One orange, or apple, or pear or 1 cup of berries.

Breakfast
One small bran muffin or 1 small oatmeal muffin with 1 teaspoon all fruit jelly or preserves.

AM Snack
Milk & Cookies: 6 ounces skim milk and 2 reduced fat fig cookies or 2 reduced fat oatmeal raisin cookies and/or calcium supplement.

Lunch
One cup salmon salad made by combining drained canned salmon, (including bones) with 1 tablespoon reduced fat mayonnaise, 2 tablespoons plain nonfat yogurt, ½ grated onion, and ¼ teaspoon pepper and served on a bed of Romaine lettuce (3 leaves) garnished with 1 sliced tomato topped with two green onions chopped fine and topped with 1 teaspoon parmesan cheese and 2 tablespoons nonfat dressing.

PM Snack
Two stalks celery stuffed with a mixture of 2 tablespoons peanut butter and 2 tablespoons calcium-enriched, low fat cottage cheese blended

Dinner
One vegetable cheese omelet made with 1 egg and 2 egg whites and ¼ cup reduced fat cheddar cheese and ¼ cup cooked broccoli & 8 asparagus spears drizzled with nonfat salad dressing.

Bedtime Snack
1 cup reduced fat frozen yogurt and/or calcium supplement.

Exercise: Today repeat yesterday. Take a 30-minute brisk walk. You can change the route to keep it interesting and fresh.

Personal Journal: Congratulations! You've completed your first week. Now compare your weight, measurements and tests from Day One and see just how much success you have achieved.

Week 2-Day 8

Pre-Breakfast
One orange, or apple, or pear or 1 cup of berries.

Breakfast
Six ounces nonfat fruit yogurt and ½ cup granola.

AM Snack
Popcorn Surprise: One cup air-popped popcorn tossed with 1
tablespoon grated parmesan cheese and/or calcium supplement.

Lunch
One cup cream of tomato soup made with skim milk and one green
salad made with 1 cup Romaine lettuce, 1 cup endive, 2 green onions
sliced, 1 tablespoon parsley, chopped tossed with 2 tablespoons nonfat
dressing.

PM Snack
Turkey Roll: Turkey roll made with 2 slices deli turkey rolled in two
large Romaine leaves.

Dinner
2 slices meatloaf or 2 hamburger patties served with large tossed salad
made with endive, romaine, tomatoes, onions, cucumbers and 2
tablespoons lowfat dressing and 1 cup steamed mixed veggies topped
with 2 teaspoons parmesan cheese.

Bedtime Snack
Bedtime Shake made with 1 cup skim milk, crushed ice and a
sprinkling of cinnamon or nutmeg and/or calcium supplement.

Exercise: Congratulations! You've done a whole week of exercise.
Now, after your 30 to 40 minute walk you can start planning to add
some weight bearing exercises.

Journal: Stay positive. Stand up straight. You'll look thinner and feel
better. Make a wish list of what you'll do when you reach your goalsl.

Week 2-Day 9

Pre-Breakfast
One orange, or apple, or pear or 1 cup of berries.

Breakfast
Breakfast Parfait made by layering 6 ounces nonfat fruit yogurt with 1 cup mixed fresh fruit such as chopped oranges, chopped apples, berries, chopped pineapple and topped with 1 tablespoon nonfat topping and 1 teaspoon chocolate sprinkles.

AM Snack
Crackers & Cheese: 4 reduced fat whole wheat crackers and 2 ounces of reduced fat cheddar or Swiss cheese and/or calcium supplement.

Lunch
One cup baked beans served with 1 cup fresh vegetables such as celery, broccoli, squash, carrots, cucumber, pea pods with ¼ cup plain nonfat yogurt flavored with pepper, and your favorite herb like basil, oregano, or rosemary, for dipping.

PM Snack
Frozen Treat: Six ounces low fat frozen yogurt, any flavor.

Dinner
Scrambled eggs made with 1 egg and 2 egg whites and served with 2 slices bacon, garnished with 1 tomato cut into wedges and topped with chopped onion and parsley and 2 tablespoons nonfat salad dressing.

Bedtime Snack
Mock Cheese Cake: 1 cup reduced fat, calcium-enriched cottage cheese topped with 1 teaspoon chopped nuts and/or calcium supplement.

Exercise: Today do a brisk walk for 30 to 45 minutes and add 15 minutes of weight bearing exercises.

Personal Journal: Today, eat your meals on a smaller plate and don't forget to nibble on the garnish—parsley is good for you.

Week 2-Day 10

Pre-Breakfast
One orange, or apple, or pear or 1 cup of berries.

Breakfast
1 cup oatmeal made with skim milk and 1 teaspoon brown sugar.

AM Snack
Sundae: 6 ounces nonfat fruit yogurt topped with ½ cup fresh berries and/or calcium supplement.

Lunch
Green salad made with one cup Romaine lettuce, 1 cup endive, 2 green onions sliced, 1 tablespoon parsley, chopped, ¼ cup croutons, 1 tablespoon parmesan cheese and 2 tablespoons nonfat dressing.

PM Snack
Spicy Cheese Snack: 2 stalks of celery stuffed with a mixture of ¼ cup calcium-enriched low fat cottage cheese and ¼ cup salsa.

Dinner
One broiled skinless, boneless chicken breast, 1 cup steamed broccoli sprinkled with 1 tablespoon parmesan cheese, 1 sliced tomato, 2 slices onion, topped with 2 tablespoons nonfat salad dressing.

Bedtime Snack
4 sticks of celery cut into 4" pieces and stuffed with 1 tablespoon peanut butter and/or calcium supplement.

Exercise: Today, try to vary your exercise. How about doing some physical work around the house? Riding a bike? Hiking?
Remember, to keep moving at a brisk pace for 30 to 60 minutes.

Personal Journal: Today clean out your kitchen pantry and toss all the foods that are high in fat, sugar and salt.

Week 2-Day 11

Pre-Breakfast
One orange, or apple, or pear or 1 cup of berries.

Breakfast
One cup calcium enriched cold cereal (Total® is a good pick) with ½ cup skim milk and topped with 1 tablespoon raisins.

AM Snack
Fruit & Cheese Plate: One orange or one apple or one pear with 1 ounce reduced fat cheddar cheese and/or calcium supplement.

Lunch
One cup calcium-enriched low fat cottage cheese topped with a mixture of 2 cups chopped fresh vegetables including zucchini, broccoli, tomato, onion, celery, cucumber and carrots and with 2 tablespoons nonfat salad dressing mixed with 2 tablespoons nonfat plain yogurt.

PM Snack
Frozen Yogurt Sundae: 6 ounces nonfat frozen vanilla yogurt topped with ½ cup blueberries or chocolate yogurt with ½ cup strawberries.

Dinner
Grilled Chicken Caesar Salad made with 2 cups Romaine lettuce, 1 teaspoon grated parmesan cheese and tossed with 2 tablespoons nonfat Caesar salad dressing and topped with 1 grilled chicken breast.

Bedtime Snack
Bedtime Shake: 1 cup skim milk, chopped ice and rum flavoring and/or calcium supplement.

Exercise: When walking today, swing your arms to get a better workout.

Personal Journal: Don't let your age impede your goals. It's just a number. Get your "body age" younger, healthier, slimmer, and more fit daily.

Week 2-Day 12

PreBreakfast
One orange, or apple, or pear or 1 cup of berries.

Breakfast
One frozen waffle toasted and topped with ¼ cup sliced strawberries mixed with ¼ cup nonfat strawberry yogurt.

AM Snack
Milk & Cookies: 6 ounces of skim milk with 2 reduced fat oatmeal cookies or 2 reduced fat fig cookies and/or calcium supplement.

Lunch
One cup low fat macaroni and cheese served with 1 cup sliced fresh vegetables such as zucchini, cucumber, broccoli, carrots served with 1 tablespoon nonfat salad dressing mixed with ¼ cup plain, nonfat yogurt for dipping.

PM Snack
A Nutty Snack: ½ cup dry roasted almonds.

Dinner
One large chef's salad made with 1 cup Romaine lettuce, 1 cup endive, 1 tomato, quartered, ½ red onion separated into rings, 1 hard boiled egg, quartered, 1 slice deli turkey cut into strips, 1 slice deli ham cut into strips, 1 ounce reduced fat cheddar and 1 ounce reduced fat Swiss cheese cut into strips and served with 2 tablespoons reduced fat salad dressing.

Bedtime Snack
1 ounce of reduced fat cheddar or swiss cheese and/or calcium supplement.

Exercise: Remember to stretch before and after your walking program for at least 5 minutes—holding each stretch for 20 seconds.

Personal Journal: Add a little spice to your life and move the salt shaker off the table today and put it away.

Week 2-Day 13

Pre-Breakfast
One orange, or apple, or pear or 1 cup of berries.

Breakfast
One bran muffin or 1 English muffin with all fruit preserves.

AM Snack
Chewy Fruit Snack: Six ounces nonfat yogurt mixed with ¼ cup chopped figs and ¼ cup raisins and/or calcium supplement.

Lunch
One baked potato topped with ¼ cup plain nonfat yogurt mixed with 1 teaspoon chopped parsley and ¼ cup salsa. One green salad with tomatoes, green onions, and reduced fat dressing.

PM Snack
Cheese & Veggie Plate: Two ounces reduced fat cheddar or Swiss cheese served on cucumber or zucchini rounds.

Dinner
Six ounces baked turkey without skin and 1 large spinach salad made with 2 cups spinach, 1 chopped tomato, 2 green onions, sliced, and garnished with ¼ cup bacon bits and 1 chopped hard-boiled egg and drizzled with 2 tablespoons nonfat salad dressing.

Bedtime Snack
Steamer: 1 cup skim milk heated and flavored with cinnamon and/or calcium supplement.

Exercise: Today you'll pick up the pace and walk faster but still keep your 30-60 minute exercise commitment.

Personal Journal: Make sure that you let a little sun shine on you today for that necessary vitamin D.

Week 2-Day 14

Pre-Breakfast
One orange, or apple, or pear or 1 cup of berries.

Breakfast
Breakfast Banana Split made with ½ cup low fat frozen vanilla yogurt, ½ small banana, ½ cup chopped orange, ½ cup chopped kiwi fruit, ½ cup raspberries.

AM Snack
Yogurt Surprise: 6 ounces nonfat vanilla yogurt topped with 1 tablespoon raisins and 1 tablespoon granola cereal and/or calcium supplement.

Lunch
One cup cream of broccoli or cream of asparagus soup made with skim milk and cantaloupe and ham wraps made by wrapping thin slices of deli ham around slices of cantaloupe. Use ½ cantaloupe and 3 slices reduced fat or nonfat deli ham.

PM Snack
Nutty Mock Cheese Cake: 6 ounces calcium-enriched, low fat cottage cheese topped 1 tablespoon chopped nuts.

Dinner
One tomato sliced and topped with 2 ounces low fat mozzarella cheese and 4 sprigs of fresh basil and one grilled hamburger patty served with 1 cup steamed spinach tossed with 2 tablespoons nonfat dressing.

Bedtime Snack
1 hard boiled egg topped with a mixture of 1 teaspoon salsa and 1 teaspoon nonfat plain yogurt and/or calcium supplement.

Exercise: Walk with a buddy. Invite a friend to walk with you today. In fact, invite several and start your own neighborhood walking club!

Personal Journal: Weigh yourself, take your measurements and re-do the Calcium Diet tests. Now compare results to Day One and Day 7. See what a success you are! Congratulations.

Week 3-Day 15

Pre-Breakfast
One orange, or apple, or pear or 1 cup of berries.

Breakfast
One cup calcium enriched cold cereal (Total® is a good pick) with ½ cup skim milk and topped with 1 tablespoon raisins.

AM Snack
Fruit & Cheese Plate: One orange or one apple or one pear with 1 ounce reduced fat cheddar cheese and/or calcium supplement.

Lunch
One cup calcium-enriched low fat cottage cheese topped with a mixture of 2 cups chopped fresh vegetables including zucchini, broccoli, tomato, onion, celery, cucumber and carrots and with 2 tablespoons nonfat salad dressing mixed with 2 tablespoons nonfat plain yogurt.

PM Snack
Frozen Yogurt Sundae: 6 ounces nonfat frozen vanilla yogurt topped with ½ cup fresh blueberries or 6 ounces nonfat frozen chocolate yogurt topped with ½ cup fresh strawberries.

Dinner
Grilled Salmon Caesar Salad made with 2 cups Romaine lettuce, 1 teaspoon grated parmesan cheese and tossed with 2 tablespoons nonfat Caesar salad dressing and topped with 1 grilled salmon steak.

Bedtime Snack
Bedtime Shake: 1 cup skim milk, chopped ice and rum flavoring and/or calcium supplement.

Exercise: Try adding light hand weights to your walk for even greater benefits.

Personal Journal: What you are is God's gift to you. What you become is your gift to God.

Week 3-Day 16

Pre-Breakfast
One orange, or apple, or pear or 1 cup of berries.

Breakfast
2 small buttermilk pancakes served with 2 teaspoons syrup.

AM Snack
Smoothie: One strawberry-banana smoothie made with 6 ounces skim milk, ½ banana and ½ cup of strawberries and/or calcium supplement.

Lunch
One small pita bread stuffed with ½ cup shredded Romaine lettuce, 1 chopped tomato, 2 sliced green onions, 2 slices of low fat cheddar cheese, sliced or shredded, ¼ cup plain nonfat yogurt and ¼ cup salsa.

PM Snack
Almond Parfait 6 ounces nonfat frozen vanilla or chocolate yogurt topped with ¼ cup chopped almonds.

Dinner
One grilled salmon or beef steak served with 1 cup coleslaw made with 1 cup shredded cabbage, ¼ cup shredded carrot, ¼ cup chopped parsley, ¼ cup nonfat yogurt, ¼ cup reduced fat mayonnaise, and one broiled tomato topped with 1 teaspoon grated parmesan cheese.

Bedtime Snack
Mock Cheesecake: 1 cup reduced fat, calcium-enriched cottage cheese topped flavored with cinnamon or nutmeg and/or calcium supplement.

Exercise: This is a good day to add some variety to your exercise program: go for a swim; hike in the country; use an exercise video.

Personal Journal: Reward yourself. Buy a new piece of clothing in your now smaller size.

Week 3-Day 17

Pre-Breakfast
One orange, or apple, or pear or 1 cup of berries.

Breakfast
One frozen waffle toasted and topped with ¼ cup sliced strawberries mixed with ¼ cup nonfat strawberry yogurt.

AM Snack
Milk & Cookies: 6 ounces of skim milk with 2 reduced fat oatmeal cookies or 2 reduced fat fig cookies and/or calcium supplement.

Lunch
One cup low fat macaroni and cheese served with 1 cup sliced fresh vegetables such as zucchini, cucumber, broccoli, carrots served with 1 tablespoon nonfat salad dressing mixed with ¼ cup plain, nonfat yogurt for dipping.

PM Snack
A Nutty Snack: ½ cup dry roasted almonds.

Dinner
One large chef's salad made with 1 cup Romaine lettuce, 1 cup endive, 1 tomato, quartered, ½ red onion separated into rings, 1 hard boiled egg, quartered, 1 slice deli turkey cut into strips, 1 slice deli ham cut into strips, 1 ounce reduced fat cheddar and 1 ounce reduced fat Swiss cheese cut into strips and 2 tablespoons reduced fat salad dressing.

Bedtime Snack
1 ounce of reduced fat cheddar or swiss cheese and/or calcium supplement.

Exercise: Increase your walking speed and your distance. Set a goal of walking a mile in 15 minutes—two miles in 30 minutes.

Personal Journal: When you shop for groceries, shop the rim of the store—that's where the fresh foods are and avoid the center aisle—that's usually where the packaged foods are.

Week 3-Day 18

Pre-Breakfast
One orange, or apple, or pear or 1 cup of berries.

Breakfast
1 cup oatmeal made with skim milk and 1 teaspoon brown sugar.

AM Snack
Sundae: 6 ounces nonfat fruit yogurt topped with ½ cup fresh berries and/or calcium supplement.

Lunch
Green salad made with one cup Romaine lettuce, 1 cup endive, 2 green onions sliced, 1 tablespoon parsley, chopped, ¼ cup croutons, 1 tablespoon parmesan cheese and 2 tablespoons nonfat dressing.

PM Snack
Spicy Cheese Snack: 2 stalks of celery stuffed with a mixture of ¼ cup calcium-enriched low fat cottage cheese and ¼ cup salsa.

Dinner
One broiled skinless, boneless chicken breast, 1 cup steamed broccoli sprinkled with 1 tablespoon parmesan cheese, 1 sliced tomato, 2 slices onion, topped with 2 tablespoons nonfat salad dressing.

Bedtime Snack
4 sticks of celery cut into 4" pieces and stuffed with 1 tablespoon peanut butter and/or calcium supplement.

Exercise: Take up a sport. Spend at least 1 hour a week practicing. Tennis, racquet ball, volley ball are good choices to start with.

Personal Journal: Make sure you get plenty of water. Try flavoring your water with fresh lemon slices.

Week 3-Day 19

Pre-Breakfast
One orange, or apple, or pear or 1 cup of berries.

Breakfast
Breakfast Banana Split made with ½ cup low fat frozen vanilla yogurt, ½ small banana, ½ cup chopped orange, ½ cup chopped kiwi fruit, ½ cup raspberries.

AM Snack
Yogurt Surprise: 6 ounces nonfat vanilla yogurt topped with 1 tablespoon raisins and 1 tablespoon granola cereal and/or calcium supplement.

Lunch
One cup cream of broccoli or cream of asparagus soup made with skim milk and cantaloupe and ham wraps made by wrapping thin slices of deli ham around slices of cantaloupe. Use ½ cantaloupe and 3 slices reduced fat or nonfat deli ham.

PM Snack
Nutty Mock Cheese Cake: 6 ounces calcium-enriched, low fat cottage cheese topped 1 tablespoon chopped nuts.

Dinner
One tomato sliced and topped with 2 ounces low fat mozzarella cheese and 4 sprigs of fresh basil and one grilled hamburger patty served with 1 cup steamed spinach tossed with 2 tablespoons nonfat dressing.

Bedtime Snack
1 hard boiled egg topped with a mixture of 1 teaspoon salsa and 1 teaspoon nonfat plain yogurt and/or calcium supplement.

Exercise: Keep it going. Remember your stretching exercises, your fat-burning exercises and your weight-bearing exercises.

Personal Journal: Look for ways to modify your favorite recipes to fit into the program on a continuing basis.

Week 3-Day 20

Pre-Breakfast
One orange, or apple, or pear or 1 cup of berries.

Breakfast
One small bagel with 1 tablespoon reduced fat cream cheese and 1 tablespoon all-fruit preserves.

AM Snack
A Taste of the Mediterranean: Five dried figs and/or calcium supplement.

Lunch
1 cup pasta topped with marinara sauce and 1 teaspoon parmesan cheese and 1 green salad made with 1 cup Romaine lettuce and 1 cup endive, ¼ cup sliced green onions, one chopped tomato, 1 sliced red or green pepper and 1 celery spine, tossed with nonfat dressing.

PM Snack
Cottage Cheese Cup: 6 ounces calcium-enriched low fat cottage cheese mixed with ½ cup fresh berries.

Dinner
One small grilled steak (4-ounces) topped with 1 cup mushrooms cooked in ¼ cup chicken broth and served with 1 cup garlic greens made with beet greens, collard greens and/or kale steamed and tossed with 1 tablespoon olive oil, 1 teaspoon minced garlic and ¼ teaspoon pepper.

Bedtime Snack
1 cup of tomato soup made with skim milk served hot or chilled and/or calcium supplement.

Exercise: Join an exercise class. There are lots of fun classes that offer something for everyone with fellowship thrown in. Become part of a group.

Personal Journal: Invest in a small food scale. That way you'll know exactly how many ounces you are eating daily.

Week 3-Day 21

Pre-Breakfast
One orange, or apple, or pear or 1 cup of berries.

Breakfast
1 frozen waffle, toasted topped with ¼ cup nonfat fruit yogurt and ¼ cup berries.

AM Snack
Fruit & Cheese Snack: One apple, one orange, or one pear and 1 ounce of reduced fat cheddar or Swiss cheese and/or calcium supplement.

Lunch
One cup cooked rice topped with broccoli stir-fry made with ½ cup broccoli florets, ½ red pepper seeded and slivered, 1 green onion, peeled and sliced thin, 1 teaspoon reduced sodium soy sauce and 1 teaspoon minced garlic cooked in 2 tablespoons chicken broth.

PM Snack
Hearty Dessert: 6 ounces calcium-enriched low fat cottage cheese mixed with ¼ cup raisins and ¼ cup chopped peanuts.

Dinner
Two cups spaghetti squash served with 1 cup tomato meat sauce made with lean ground beef, topped with 1 tablespoon grated parmesan cheese and 1 green salad made with 1 cup romaine lettuce, 1 cup endive, 1 tomato, 2 green onions, tossed with 2 tablespoons nonfat salad dressing.

Bedtime Snack
2 stalks celery cut into 4" pieces and stuffed with a mixture of peanut butter and reduced fat, calcium-enriched cottage cheese, blended smooth and/or calcium supplement.

Exercise: Congratulations! Now keep it going.

Personal Journal: Take all your measurements and re-do the tests today. Now compare the after you, with the before you. Keep it up. God bless!

Chapter 13   The Non-Dairy Calcium Diet for the Dairy Challenged

I think you should know, that most of the studies on the effect of calcium on weight and fat loss have been done on lowfat dairy derived sources of calcium, and calcium supplements.

And experts all agree, that dairy products are one of the best sources of dietary calcium because of the other nutrients contained in the mix—vitamins and other nutrients.

There is a very real issue, however, of lactose intolerance and milk allergy. You should check with your own health care provider to determine whether or not you suffer from one of these and what treatments can be implemented.

If you find that you simply cannot tolerate dairy products, or don't like them, or object to them on any other grounds, there are non-dairy sources of calcium that can help to fill your daily requirements.

Make sure that you do get some calcium from your food, and then ask your health care provider about supplementing with calcium supplements to make sure you have adequate amounts daily.

Here is a guide to help you plan your non-dairy based *Calcium Diet*. Enjoy!

Non-Dairy Calcium Diet Week 1-Day 1

Pre-Breakfast
One orange, or apple, or pear or 1 cup of berries.

Breakfast
One frozen waffle with 1 tablespoon all-fruit spread.

AM Snack
1 frozen waffle with ½ cup berries. One calcium supplement.

Lunch
One cup baked beans with one side salad made with 1 cup romaine lettuce, 1 cup endive, 2 sliced green onions, and one tomato tossed with 2 tablespoons nonfat dressing.

PM Snack
½ cup dried figs.

Dinner
Grilled salmon (6-ounces) served with 1 cup steamed broccoli, ½ cup collards and 1 grilled tomato.

Bedtime Snack
3 slices deli ham and 1 hard boiled egg. One calcium supplement.

Exercise: Today begin your exercise program by writing down your exercise goals—30 to 60 minutes of exercise per day;

Personal Journal: Write in your starting weight, your measurements and the results of the three Calcium Diet tests.

Non-Dairy Calcium Diet Week 1-Day 2
Pre-Breakfast
One orange, or apple, or pear or 1 cup of berries.

Breakfast
2 small pancakes and 1 teaspoon all-fruit preserves.

AM Snack
Fruit & Sweets Snack: 1 medium apple and 2 fig cookies. Calcium supplement.

Lunch
One small baked potato topped with ½ cup steamed collard greens mixed with ¼ cup salsa and 1 tablespoon chopped parsley.

PM Snack
1 can sardines with bones served on cucumber and zucchini rounds.

Dinner
1 steak (6 ounces) with 1 cup mixed greens (mustard, collard, beet) flavored with a squeeze of lemon juice and one salad made with 1 cup Romaine, 1 cup endive, 1 chopped tomato, 2 green onions, sliced thin, tossed with 2 tablespoons nonfat salad dressing.

Bedtime Snack
3 slices deli turkey and 1 tomato. Calcium supplement.

Exercise: Today get a check-up to make sure that you are in shape to begin an exercise program if you haven't exercised for a long time and are out of shape. When you get an O.K. from your own doctor, you are ready to begin.

Personal Journal: Make a note beside each meal that you ate today and any "extras".

Non-Dairy Calcium Diet Week 1-Day 3

Pre-Breakfast
One orange, or apple, or pear or 1 cup of berries.

Breakfast
One toasted English muffin and 1 tablespoon all-fruit spread.

AM Snack
½ cup dried figs. Calcium supplement.

Lunch
One glass (6-ounces) tomato juice and one veggie wrap made with 1 corn tortilla, ½ cup shredded romaine lettuce, 1 chopped tomato, ½ cup shredded spinach, 2 green onions, chopped, 1 tablespoon chopped parsley and ¼ cup tofu mixed with ¼ cup salsa.

PM Snack
1 can (3 ¾ ounces) salmon with bones mixed served with ½ cup raw broccoli florets.

Dinner
Grilled salmon (6-ounces) served with 1 cup steamed broccoli and 1 green salad made with 1 cup Romaine lettuce, 1 cup endive, 1 tomato, 2 green onions, 2 teaspoons chopped parsley, ½ cup cucumber, ½ cup radishes and drizzled with 2 tablespoons nonfat salad dressing.

Bedtime Snack
1 small omelet made with 1 egg and 1 egg white. Calcium supplement

Exercise: Today is your prep day. Schedule time in your day for exercise. Make sure your exercise clothing is in good shape.

Personal Journal: Make notes today about your weight—remember to weigh yourself at the same time and congratulate yourself for being motivated to begin a program of weight management and better health.

Non Dairy Calcium Diet Week 1-Day 4
Pre-Breakfast
One orange, or apple, or pear or 1 cup of berries.

Breakfast
1 bran muffin and ½ cup raisins

AM Snack
1 frozen waffle topped with 1 tablespoon all-fruit spread and ½ cup dried figs. Calcium supplement.

Lunch
½ cup baked beans and a green salad made with 1 cup Romaine lettuce, 1 cup endive, 2 green onions sliced, 1 tablespoon parsley, chopped and 2 tablespoons nonfat dressing.

PM Snack
¼ cup mixed nuts such as peanuts and almonds.

Dinner
Grilled chicken breast served with 1 cup steamed broccoli, 1 cup steamed greens such as collard and 1 sliced tomato, 2 slices onion, topped with 2 tablespoons nonfat salad dressing

Bedtime Snack
1 tomato stuffed with 1 individual can (3 ¾ ounces) salmon with bones. Calcium supplement.

Exercise: Post your exercise intentions on your dashboard, the fridge, on the side of your computer, your bathroom mirror—anywhere you can to be reminded about your good intentions to begin. Exercise motivation is your key, today.

Personal Journal: Keep up with your food entries and remember, every day you are getting slimmer and healthier.

Non Dairy Calcium Diet Week 1-Day 5

Pre-Breakfast
One orange, or apple, or pear or 1 cup of berries.

Breakfast
2 small pancakes with 2 teaspoons all-fruit preserves.

AM Snack
1 medium apple and ½ cup dried figs. Calcium supplement.

Lunch
One small baked potato topped with ¼ cup tofu mixed with ¼ cup salsa
and 1 tablespoon chopped parsley.

PM Snack
¼ cup dry roasted almonds

Dinner
Six ounces mackerel, baked or broiled served with 1 cup mixed greens
flavored with a squeeze of lemon juice and one salad made with 1 cup
Romaine, 1 cup endive, 1 chopped tomato, 2 green onions, sliced thin,
tossed with 2 tablespoons nonfat salad dressing.

Bedtime Snack
3 slices deli turkey. Calcium supplement.

Exercise: Time to get started. The Centers for Disease Control
recommend that you keep a pair of good walking shoes in your car so
that you'll always be ready to start walking. Today, your goal is to walk
for 10 minutes—twice between breakfast and bedtime.

Personal Journal: Record your weight today, the foods you ate and
your growing positive feeling about yourself.

Non-Dairy Calcium Diet Week 1-Day 6

Pre-Breakfast
One orange, or apple, or pear or 1 cup of berries.

Breakfast
2 waffles with 2 teaspoons all-fruit spread 1 cup berries.

AM Snack
Popcorn Surprise: One cup air-popped popcorn tossed with 1 tablespoon of your favorite herb or spice. Calcium supplement.

Lunch
One cup baked beans and one green salad made with 1 cup Romaine lettuce, 1 cup endive, 2 green onions sliced, 1 tablespoon parsley, chopped tossed with 2 tablespoons nonfat dressing.

PM Snack
Turkey Roll: Turkey roll made with 2 slices deli turkey rolled in two large Romaine leaves.

Dinner
A veggie omelet made with 2 eggs and 1 egg white and 1 cup cooked broccoli and served with 1 cup green beans topped with 1 tablespoon sliced almonds.

Bedtime Snack
½ cup tofu-type frozen dessert. One calcium supplement.
.

Exercise: Today increase your walking from 10 minutes twice a day to 15 minutes twice a day. Try to increase your pace, too. How about walking in the mall? Walking around the block? Walking to the store and back?

Personal Journal: Record your weight and your meals and remember you CAN reach your goals. You are not alone.

Non-Dairy Calcium Diet Week 1-Day 7

Pre-Breakfast
One orange, or apple, or pear or 1 cup of berries.

Breakfast
One small bran muffin or 1 small oatmeal muffin with 1 teaspoon all fruit jelly or preserves.

AM Snack
2 oatmeal cookies and ½ cup dried figs and ¼ cantaloupe. Calcium supplement.

Lunch
One cup salmon salad made by combining drained canned salmon, (including bones) with 1 tablespoon reduced fat mayonnaise, ¼ cup tablespoons plain tofu, ½ grated onion, and ¼ teaspoon pepper and served on a bed of Romaine lettuce (3 leaves) garnished with 1 sliced tomato topped with two green onions chopped fine and 2 tablespoons nonfat dressing.

PM Snack
Two stalks celery stuffed with a mixture of 2 tablespoons peanut butter and 2 tablespoons tofu blended

Dinner
One salmon steak (6 ounces) with 1 cup steamed greens and 8 asparagus spears drizzled with nonfat salad dressing.

Bedtime Snack
3 slices deli turkey and 1 sliced tomato. Calcium supplement.

Exercise: Today repeat yesterday. Take a 30-minute brisk walk. You can change the route to keep it interesting and fresh.

Personal Journal: Congratulations! You've completed your first week. Now compare your weight, measurements and tests from Day One and see just how much success you have achieved.

Menu Suggestions for Non-Dairy Calcium Diet

Pre-Breakfast
Orange, apple, pear or 1 cup of berries

Breakfast
Waffles, pancakes, breads, muffins, dry cereals. All-fruit spreads.

Morning Snacks
2 fig cookies, ½ cup dried figs, 2 oatmeal cookies, ¼ cup raisins, 1 cup air-popped popcorn, muffin, waffle, pancake, 1 slice bread, muffin

Lunch
½ cup baked beans, corn tortilla, steamed greens, collard, mustard, beet, Romaine and endive salad, canned salmon, tofu omelet

Afternoon Snacks
Hard boiled eggs, deli meats such as sliced turkey, ham, roast beef, canned salmon or sardines with bones, ¼ cup dry roasted nuts, Tofu-type dessert

Dinner
Chicken breast, turkey, steak, grilled salmon or mackerel, or omelets, collard or other greens, salad made with Romaine and/or endive

Bedtime Snacks
Deli meats, Tofu-type desserts, hard-boiled eggs.

Note: for a more complete list of non-dairy based calcium foods please refer to the Resources section.

Chapter 14

The Calcium Diet
& Other Diets

This chapter is about calcium and how it can help you achieve the goals you hope for with whatever diet or food plan or weight management program is your favorite.

I believe that *The Calcium Diet* is a wonderful SOLO plan—the only plan you'll need to achieve your weight loss, fitness and health goals.

But one of the most exciting and special features of *The Calcium Diet* is its unique ability to work with whatever your favorite program is and help you to reach your goals successfully. Perhaps you've been following a favorite program and have reached a plateau. Perhaps you are stuck. Perhaps you are discouraged. Bored. Frustrated. But, you don't want to leave a program that you like and that has been successful for you in the past. Now you can give yourself a fat burning boost by adding additional calcium to your favorite diet plan, either through dairy foods, non-dairy foods, or calcium supplements.

When you add food sources of calcium to your favorite diet program, either through dairy or non-dairy sources, be careful not to change the integrity of the author's program. If you aren't sure whether adding additional dietary sources of calcium either through dairy or non-dairy foods will change or alter the integrity of the program, then consider adding calcium supplements morning and night to bring the total level of calcium to a fat fighting level recommended in this book.

A good rule of thumb regarding food that is calcium-rich, is to try to use nonfat yogurt in place of sour cream and/or mayonnaise; to select fish, such as salmon, and sardines that are high in calcium, whenever you have a fish or protein choice; to add greens such as mustard greens, collard greens, beet greens to any mixed vegetables and to focus on such high calcium veggies as broccoli. To experiment with tofu and marine vegetables which are also high in calcium.

Finally, remember, that you may be particularly vulnerable to a calcium deficiency when you are dieting and that it may be necessary to add calcium morning and night as a supplement to make sure that you are getting the recommended amounts for health and to help your body reach the weight and health goals you have set.

Here is a list of the most popular diets and weight-loss programs that you could add calcium to, in order to boost their fat fighting power with the breakthrough power of calcium.

Dieting With The Duchess
Dr. Atkins' New Diet Revolution
Eat More Weigh Less
Eat Right 4 Your Type
Edita's Skinny System
Fit For Life
Jenny Craig's What Have You Got To Lose?
Protein Power
The 5 Day Miracle Diet
The Business Plan for the Body
The Fat Flush Plan
The New Sugar Busters
The Schwarzbein Principle
The South Beach Diet
The Starch Blocker Diet
The Weigh Down Diet
The Zone

Part Four

The Recipes Part

Blueberry Yogurt Muffins

1 ½ cups wheat bran
½ cup boiling water
1 ⅓ cups whole-wheat flour
1 ¼ cups baking soda
½ teaspoon ground cinnamon
¼ teaspoon ground cloves
¼ teaspoon ground nutmeg
1 egg
⅓ cup honey
3 tablespoons vegetable oil
½ cup plain, nonfat yogurt
¾ cups blueberries, fresh or frozen

Preheat oven to 350°
1. Line muffin tins with paper baking cups.
2. In a medium bowl combine the wheat bran and boiling water. Let stand 10 minutes to soften.
3. In a small bowl combine the egg, honey, yogurt and oil. Stir well. Add to the bran mixture.
4. In a large bowl combine the flour, baking soda, and spices.
5. Add the egg mixture to the flour mixture all at once. Stir until the dry ingredients are moistened. The batter will be stiff. Fold in the blueberries.
6. Fill prepared muffin cups ⅔ full. Bake 20 to 25 minutes or until toothpick inserted in the center comes out clean. Serve warm.

Makes: 12 muffins
Calories: 138

Serving size: 1 muffin
Calcium: 33 mg

Mediterranean Muffins

1 ½ cups all-purpose flour
2 tablespoons sugar
1 tablespoon baking powder
2 cups bran flakes cereal
1 ¼ cups orange juice
2 egg whites
2 tablespoons vegetable oil
1 cup chopped dried figs
1 teaspoon grated orange peel

Preheat oven to 400°F.
1. Line muffin tins with paper baking cups.
2. Stir together the flour, sugar and baking powder. Set aside.
3. Mix together the cereal, orange juice, egg, oil, figs, and orange peel. Mix until well blended.
4. Add the dry ingredients to the cereal mixture. Stir until just combined.
5. Fill muffin cups ⅔ full. Bake for 25 minutes or until golden brown. Serve warm.

Makes 12 muffins   Serving size: 1 muffin
Calories: 164   Calcium: 116 mg

Edita's Tip: Dried figs are a wonderful source of calcium and make a terrific snack all by themselves.Try them.

Mountain Muesli

1 cup rolled oats
½ cup raisins
2 cups plain, nonfat yogurt
2 tablespoons honey
1 cup apples, cored and sliced thin

1. In a large bowl combine rolled oats, raisins, and yogurt. Stir until well combined. Cover and refrigerate overnight.
2. Top with fresh apples and drizzle with honey before serving. Serve chilled.

Makes 4 servings
Calories: 244

Serving size: ½ cup
Calcium: 248 mg

Edita's Tip: This is a wonderful dish to keep in the fridge for breakfast. Try it with different fruit on top. Thinly sliced pears, strawberries, or raspberries. You can also toss in some finely chopped dried figs to give yourself an even bigger calcium boost.

Hot Apple Spice Oatmeal

1 apple, cored, unpeeled and chopped
⅔ cup rolled oats
1 cup skim milk
½ teaspoon cinnamon

1. Put the milk, apple and rolled oats into a medium saucepan and bring to a boil.
2. Reduce heat and simmer until oatmeal thickens, stirring constantly. Stir in cinnamon. Serve hot.

Makes 2 servings
Calories 189

Serving size: ½ cup
Calcium 177 mg

Edita's Tip: Try this with other fruit. I find it tastes delicious with pears, raisins, or fresh or frozen blueberries.

Farm Fresh Buttermilk Pancakes

1 cup flour
1 teaspoon sugar
¾ teaspoon baking powder
½ teaspoon baking soda
1 egg or egg substitute equivalent
1 cup buttermilk
1 tablespoon liquid Butter Buds®
vegetable cooking spray

1. Sift together the flour, sugar, baking powder, and baking soda.
2. Beat egg lightly. Add the buttermilk and Butter Buds to the egg.
3. Add the egg mixture to the dry ingredients.
4. Spray a nonstick skillet with vegetable cooking spray. Heat. Pour batter into hot skillet making pancakes of approximately 4-inches in diameter. Fry on both sides until golden. Serve hot.

Makes 10 pancakes
Calories: 220

Serving size: 2 pancakes
Calcium: 132 mg

Edita's Tip: Try a glass of chilled buttermilk as a way of getting your daily dairy calcium requirement. It's particularly refreshing on a hot summer afternoon.

Spicy Muffins

2 cups all-purpose
3 tablespoons sugar
1 ½ tablespoons baking powder
½ teaspoon cinnamon
¼ cup liquid Butter Buds®
1 cup skim milk
1 egg white

Preheat oven to 425°F.
1. Line muffin tins with paper baking cups.
2. In a small bowl, combine the milk and oil.
3. Add the Butter Buds and milk to the dry mixture. Stir gently until just combined.
4. Beat the egg white until stiff peaks form. Fold the beaten egg white into the mixture.
5. Fill the prepared muffin cups ⅔ full. Bake for 20 minutes or until a toothpick inserted in the center comes out clean.

Makes 12 servings   Serving size: 1 muffin
Calories: 106   Calcium: 131 mg

Edita's Tip: Why not make an extra batch and toss them into the freezer. Then throw a couple into your car, or gym bag or briefcase for a wonderful AM snack.

Baked Breakfast Apples

4 large apples, cored and sliced
1 teaspoon cinnamon
4 tablespoons brown sugar
2 cups plain nonfat yogurt

Preheat oven to 375°F
   1. Spray a nonstick casserole with cooking spray.
   2. Arrange the apple slices in the bottom of the casserole. Top with cinnamon and brown sugar.
   3. Bake, uncovered for 30 to 40 minutes or until apples are tender.
   4. Transfer to serving dishes and top with equal amounts of the yogurt.

Makes 4 servings
Calories: 180   Calcium: 250 mg

Edita's Tip: I love these either hot or cold and often pack a portion in a little plastic container to enjoy as a snack at my desk or on the go.

Breakfast On The Run

1 cup granola
1 cup low fat yogurt, any flavor

Stir cereal into the yogurt. Serve.

Makes 4 servings
Calories: 184   Calcium: 123 mg

Edita's Tip: Again, this makes a great morning or afternoon snack and the variety is endless. Just mix any good, low fat granola with any low fat yogurt—even the ones with fruit. If you pack a little granola in a plastic bag and keep it in the car or in your desk, you'll always be able to make this healthy and satisfying snack.

Chocolate Breakfast Whip

1 cup skim milk
1 cup skim milk powder
1 teaspoon instant coffee
2 teaspoons cocoa
1 tablespoon sugar
8 ice cubes

Put all ingredients into a blender or food processor and process until smooth. Serve.

Makes 4 servings
Calories: 144   Calcium: 455 mg

Edita's Tip: If you are a true lover of chocolate, you will really enjoy this breakfast. And guess what? It makes a great chocolate snack whenever you need a little chocolate indulgence.

Breakfast Rice Pudding

1 cup regular long grain rice
4 cups skim milk
½ cup sugar
2 teaspoons vanilla extract

Preheat oven to 325° F
1. In a small saucepan combine the rice, milk, sugar and vanilla. Simmer uncovered for 5 to 7 minutes.
2. Turn mixture into a nonstick 2-quart baking dish coated with cooking spray. Cover lightly with foil. Bake 30 to 40 minutes or until all the liquid has been absorbed.
3. Remove from oven. Serve warm.

Makes 6 servings
Calories: 238   Calcium: 210 mg

Edita's Tip: Try a few drops of lemon extract instead of the vanilla, or rum. How about a few drops of food coloring? Pink rice pudding for breakfast!

Orange-Raspberry Breakfast Trifle

4 ounces nonfat cream cheese
4 ounces nonfat ricotta cheese
2 cups raspberries
4 oranges, peeled and sliced
¼ cup raspberry jam
¼ cup orange marmalade
16 vanilla wafers, crumbled
1 container (8-ounces) low fat vanilla yogurt

1. Place the cheeses into a blender or food processor. Process until smooth.
2. In a separate bowl combine the raspberry jam and orange marmalade. Add ½ the raspberries and ½ the oranges to the jam and marmalade mixture.
3. Assemble the trifle in a large bowl in layers as follows: first layer cheese mixture. Next fruit and jam mixture. Next vanilla wafers. Next a layer of raspberries and a layer of oranges.
4. Chill for 2 hours. Serve topped with large dollop of vanilla yogurt.

Makes 8 servings
Calories: 200   Calcium: 174 mg

Hawaiian Snack Mix

4 cups Total® cereal
¼ cup brown sugar
¼ cup liquid Butter Buds®
1 tablespoon grated orange peel
1 cup dried pineapple pieces
½ cup banana chips
½ cup flaked coconut

Preheat oven to 300°F
1. Place cereal in a nonstick baking pan
2. In a nonstick saucepan heat the sugar and Butter Buds over low heat. Stir in the orange peel.
3. Pour mixture over the cereal. Toss until evenly coated. Bake 20 minutes, stirring twice.
4. Stir in the remaining ingredients.
5. Cool. Store in airtight container.

Makes: 16 servings
Calories: 147   Calcium: 64 mg approx

Southwestern Snack

3 cups Total® cereal
3 cups hot-air popped popcorn
1 cup cheese crackers
1 cup pretzel sticks
1 tablespoon vegetable oil
½ teaspoon chili powder
¼ teaspoon ground cumin
½ teaspoon garlic powder
¼ cup Parmesan cheese, grated

Preheat oven to 300°F

1. Mix all the ingredients together in a large plastic bag. Shake to coat well.
2. Pour into a nonstick baking pan. Bake 10 minutes without stirring.
3. Cool. Store in a tightly covered container.

Makes: 24 servings
Calories: 89   Calcium: 53 mg approx

Roman Crostini

¼ cup fresh basil, chopped fine
¼ cup fresh parsley, chopped fine
2 tablespoons white wine
2 tablespoons lemon juice
1 teaspoon olive oil
8 slices Italian bread, sliced into ¼-inch thick slices
4 tablespoons goat cheese
2 tomatoes, sliced into 8 thick slices
½ teaspoon black pepper
½ teaspoon coarse salt

Preheat oven to 350ºF
1. Place the basil, parsley, wine, lemon juice and olive oil into a blender or food processor and process until smooth.
2. Place the bread slices on a nonstick cookie sheet and bake for 5 to 7 minutes or until crisp.
3. Spread each slice of bread with an even amount of the cheese.
4. Top each slice with a slice of tomato and drizzle with the herb mixture. Finish with salt and pepper.

Makes: 8 servings
Calories: 86   Calcium: 55 mg

Spicy Potato Wedges

½ cup all-purpose flour
½ cup Parmesan cheese, grated
4 baking potatoes, scrubbed and cut each into 8 wedges
½ cup skim milk powder
¼ cup margarine, melted
1 teaspoon paprika
1 teaspoon coarse salt
½ teaspoon pepper
½ teaspoon garlic powder

Preheat oven to 400°F
1. Place all the ingredients into a large plastic bag. Seal and shake until the potatoes are coated.
2. Arrange the potato wedges on a nonstick cookie sheet sprayed with cooking spray. Bake for 20 minutes.
3. Turn and bake 20 minutes more or until golden and tender. Serve.

Makes: 8 servings
Calories: 204   Calcium: 176 mg

Edita's Tip: Try serving these with a little plain nonfat yogurt mixed with your favorite seasonings for a great dip.

Golden Melon Smoothie

½ cantaloupe, peeled and seeded
1 cup skim milk
1 cup plain, nonfat yogurt
1 cup crushed ice
2 to 4 packets artificial sweetener

Place all ingredients in a blender. Process until smooth.
Serve.

Makes: 2 servings
Calories: 162   Calcium: 395 mg

Tropical Smoothie

1 mango, peeled and sliced
1 kiwi fruit, peeled and sliced
1 banana, peeled and sliced
1 cup frozen strawberries
1 container (8-ounces) low fat strawberry banana yogurt
2 cups skim milk

Place all ingredients into a blender. Process until smooth.
Serve.

Makes: 4 servings
Calories: 216   Calcium: 271 mg

Fruit Cocktail Frosty

1 can (16 ounces) fruit cocktail in juice, undrained
½ cup skim milk powder
1 teaspoon vanilla extract
1 cup crushed ice

Combine all ingredients in a blender. Process until smooth.
Serve.

Makes: 2 servings
Calories: 219   Calcium: 397 mg

Café au Lait

½ cup coffee, brewed strong, hot
½ cup skim milk, hot

Pour hot coffee and hot milk into cup at the same time.
Serve.

Makes: 1 serving
Calories: 45   Calcium: 154

Edita's Tip: This is my favorite Saturday morning coffee.
But don't overdo it…this drink still contains caffeine.

Peach Frosty

1 can (16 ounces) peach slices in juice, undrained
½ cup skim milk powder
1 teaspoon vanilla extract
1 cup crushed ice

Combine all ingredients in a blender. Process until smooth. Serve.

Makes: 2 servings
Calories: 215   Calcium: 393

Strawberry Slush

1 package (10-ounces) frozen strawberries, thawed
1 cup skim milk
2 cups nonfat frozen yogurt, vanilla or strawberry

Place all ingredients into a blender and process until smooth. Serve.

Makes: 4 servings
Calories: 155   Calcium: 180 mg

Almond Smoothie

1 container (8 ounces) lowfat peach yogurt
1 cup sliced peaches, frozen
½ teaspoon almond extract

Place all ingredients into a blender and process until smooth. Serve.

Makes 4 servings
Calories: 37   Calcium: 104

Fruit & Veggie Calcium Cocktail

4 carrots, scrubbed
2 apples, cored

In a juicer, liquefy all ingredients. Serve.

Makes: 2 servings
Calories: 143   Calcium: 49 mg

Berry Calcium Cocktail

1 cup cranberries, fresh or frozen
2 apples, cored
1 orange, peeled and sectioned

In a juicer, liquefy all ingredients. Serve.

Makes: 2 servings
Calories: 135   Calcium: 39 mg

Russian Potato Salad Platter

2 pounds potatoes, peeled, cooked, diced
1 onion, peeled and chopped fine
4 mushrooms, sliced thin
1 container (8-ounces) plain, nonfat yogurt
3 tablespoons chives, chopped
½ teaspoon salt
¼ teaspoon pepper

1. Spray a nonstick skillet with cooking spray and sauté the onion and mushroom, cooking until the juices run.
2. Add the potatoes, salt, pepper and chives and brown. Turn over and brown on the other side.
3. Add the yogurt and mix gently until all the ingredients are coated. Heat the mixture. Serve.

Makes: 4 servings
Calories: 216   Calcium: 134 mg

Edita's Tip: Try sprinkling a little chopped dill on this salad and serve it on a big leaf of dark green Romaine lettuce with chunks of fresh tomato, slivers of celery, cucumber rounds and any other of your favorite veggies. It's a meal in itself.

Macaroni Salad

2 cups elbow macaroni, cooked
1 cup baby peas, frozen and thawed
1 cup green olives stuffed with pimentos, sliced thin
1 red onion, peeled and chopped fine
2 stalks celery with tops, chopped fine
1 green pepper, seeded and diced
1 red pepper, seeded and diced
2 teaspoons dry mustard
½ cup fat free mayonnaise
½ cup fat free sour cream
¼ cup skim milk powder
½ teaspoon salt
¼ teaspoon pepper

Combine all ingredients in a large bowl. Mix well. Serve.

Makes: 8 servings
Calories: 136   Calcium: 87 mg

Edita's Tip: This is a wonderful picnic salad—even if your picnic is in your own living room. Spread out a checkered cloth. Arrange some flowers. And you and your family can enjoy this meal together any time of the year.

Corn Chowder

2 tablespoons liquid Butter Buds®
1 onion, peeled and chopped
1 red pepper, seeded and chopped fine
1 green pepper, seeded and chopped fine
1 tablespoon all-purpose flour
2 cups skim milk
1 can (8-ounces) corn kernels, drained
1 tablespoon dried thyme
¼ teaspoon pepper

1. In a medium nonstick saucepan sprayed with cooking spray cook the onion and peppers until soft, stirring often, about 5 minutes.
2. Add flour, stirring constantly about 1 minute.
3. Gradually add the milk, corn, Butter Buds, thyme and pepper. Reduce heat to low. Cook 5 minutes more or until slightly thickened. Serve.

Makes: 4 servings
Calories: 137   Calcium: 185 mg

Edita's Tip: Many soups can be calcium-enhanced with a spoonful of nonfat powdered skim milk. It adds calcium and creaminess.

Creamy Potato Soup

1 tablespoon margarine
1 onion, peeled and chopped fine
¼ cup celery, chopped fine
1 large potato, peeled and chopped fine
1 cup chicken broth
¼ cup parsley, chopped fine
¼ teaspoon dried thyme
¼ teaspoon white pepper
1 ½ cups skim milk

1. Melt the margarine in a medium, nonstick saucepan over medium-high heat.
2. Add onion and celery and cook, stirring often, until soft.
3. Add potatoes, broth, parsley and spices. Bring to a boil. Reduce heat. Cover and simmer until potatoes are tender. Reduce heat to low.
4. Add milk. Simmer uncovered for 5 minutes.
5. Pour the mixture into a blender or food processor. Process until smooth.
6. Return to saucepan and heat through. Serve.

Makes: 4 servings
Calories: 92   Calcium: 134 mg

Winter Cabbage Soup

1 medium head cabbage, shredded fine
1 onion, peeled and sliced thin
1 carrot, peeled and sliced thin
1 celery stalk, sliced thin
1 potato, peeled and sliced thin
2 cups skim milk
1 container (8-ounces) plain, nonfat yogurt
1 bay leaf
½ teaspoon dill
¼ teaspoon pepper

1. Place the vegetables in a large nonstick saucepan. Add water until just covered.
2. Cover and simmer until vegetables are tender. About 12 to 15 minutes.
3. Add the milk, yogurt and spices. Simmer another 10 minutes. Do not allow soup to boil. Serve.

Makes: 6 servings
Calories: 83   Calcium: 196 mg

Edita's Tip: This soup is wonderful served with thick slices of fresh rye bread or pumpernickel. It's full of vitamins and gives you a wonderful satisfied feeling.

Sherry Crab Bisque

1 onion, peeled and chopped fine
1 stalk celery, chopped fine
1 carrot, peeled and chopped fine
1 potato, peeled and diced
1 can (14-ounces) chicken broth
1 can (14-ounces) cream of potato soup
¼ teaspoon dried thyme
¼ teaspoon white pepper
1 tablespoon tomato paste
1 tablespoon Worcestershire sauce
6 ounces lump crabmeat
¼ cup dry sherry
1 cup skim milk
¼ cup parsley, chopped fine
¼ cup chives, chopped fine

1. Combine the onion, celery, carrot, potato, and chicken broth, potato soup in a large, nonstick saucepan and bring to a boil.
2. Reduce heat and simmer until vegetables are tender, about 10 minutes.
3. Add the spices, crabmeat, milk and sherry. Heat through.
4. Transfer the soup to a blender or food processor. Process until smooth.
5. Return to saucepan and heat through. Serve garnished with fresh parsley and fresh chives.

Makes: 8 servings
Calories: 89   Calcium: 79 mg

Texas Potato Topper

1 cup plain nonfat yogurt
⅓ cup salsa, mild or medium, chunky style
⅓ cup stuffed green olive, chopped fine
2 baked potatoes

1. In a small bowl combine all the ingredients.
2. Cover. Chill until ready to serve.
3. Top baked potatoes with the mixture.

Makes: 2 servings
Calories: 198   Calcium: 267 mg

Edita's Tip: Try different types of salsa with this recipe. If
you want, you can also skip the olives and chop in some
extra fresh cucumber, radish, or even some extra tomatoes
are delicious with this recipe.

Quick Cheese & Tomato Rice Melt

1 cup rice
½ cup reduced fat cheddar cheese, shredded
1 cup condensed tomato soup
1. In a nonstick saucepan cook rice according to
   package directions.
2. When the rice is almost done, add the cheese and
   tomato soup. Stir until combined and the cheese
   melts. Serve hot.

Makes: 6 servings
Calories: 85   Calcium: 47 mg

Cheese Stuffed Potato Shells

4 potatoes, baked
1 cup reduced fat cottage cheese
½ cup skim milk
1 onion, minced
1 tablespoon parsley, chopped fine
¼ teaspoon pepper
½ teaspoon salt

Preheat oven to 350°F
1. Cut potatoes lengthwise and scoop out leaving shells intact.
2. Transfer the potato to a blender or food processor.
3. Add the cottage cheese, milk, onion, and ½ the parsley and the salt and pepper. Process until smooth.
4. Spoon mixture back into the potato shells.
5. Bake until golden, about 30 minutes. Sprinkle remaining parsley on each potato. Serve hot.

Makes: 8 servings
Calories: 137   Calcium: 51 mg

Edita's Tip: Try adding different herbs and spices to this dish for a different taste sensation each time. Again, remember to use the calcium-enriched cottage cheese for the most calcium benefit.

Creamy Macaroni & Cheese

1 package (8-ounces) elbow macaroni
2 cups cheddar cheese, reduced fat, shredded
1 ½ cups evaporated skim milk
¼ teaspoon white pepper

Preheat oven to 350°F
1. Cook macaroni according to package directions. Drain.
2. Add the cheese, milk and pepper. Mix well.
3. Turn into a nonstick casserole sprayed with cooking spray. Bake for 30 minutes or until heated through stirring occasionally. Serve hot.

Makes: 6 servings
Calories: 256   Calcium: 349 mg

Edita's Tip: To get even more calcium punch out of this American favorite toss a spoonful or two of dry powdered skim milk into the dish when you mix it up. Serve this with juicy wedges of fresh tomato, crunchy celery, and fresh broccoli florets.

Garlicky Mashed Potato Lunch

1 tablespoon olive oil
1 clove garlic, peeled and minced
4 cups water
4 potatoes, peeled, cut into quarters
1 cup plain nonfat yogurt
¼ cup skim milk
¼ cup scallions or green onions, chopped fine
¼ teaspoon black pepper

1. In a large, nonstick saucepan sauté the garlic in the olive oil until soft, about 1 minute.
2. Add the water and potatoes. Cover. Bring to a boil. Reduce heat and simmer 15-20 minutes until potatoes are tender. Drain.
3. Return potatoes to the saucepan. Add yogurt and milk. Mash and stir until creamy.
4. Stir in the scallions and pepper. Serve hot.

Makes: 6 servings
Calories: 111   Calcium: 101 mg

Edita's Tip: I love to heap this on dark green leaves of Romaine or even stuff stalks of celery with my mashed potatoes. It's a really terrific dish if you just really crave potatoes.

Super Spinach Salad

4 cups spinach leaves, washed, dried, torn into bits
½ head Romaine lettuce, washed, and dried, torn into bits
¼ pound mushrooms, sliced thin
1 large tomato, cut into wedges
1 onion, peeled and sliced thin
½ cup feta cheese, crumbled
1 cup buttermilk
½ cup plain, nonfat yogurt
¼ cup reduced fat Italian salad dressing
1 tablespoon white vinegar
1 teaspoon dill
1 clove garlic, peeled and chopped fine
1 teaspoon Dijon-type mustard
½ teaspoon salt
¼ teaspoon pepper

In a large salad bowl, combine all ingredients, tossing
lightly until well coated. Chill for 2 hours. Serve.

Makes: 4 servings
Calories: 154   Calcium: 304 mg

Edita's Tip: Remember, while spinach is fairly high in
calcium, that calcium is not readily absorbed. But there are
so many other wonderful nutrients in spinach that it
deserves a salad of its very own.

Italian Antipasto

2 red peppers, roasted, skinned and halved
½ pound part skim Mozzarella, cut into four slices
8 sardines in tomato sauce
8 black olives
1 tablespoon olive oil
2 tablespoons parsley, chopped fine
1 lemon cut into wedges
4 large Romaine lettuce leaves
¼ teaspoon black pepper

1. Arrange the red peppers on four small plates, which have a Romaine lettuce leaf on each.
2. Place a slice of Mozzarella on each red pepper. Arrange two sardines on the cheese.
3. Drizzle with olive oil. Sprinkle with pepper and parsley. Garnish with lemon wedges.

Makes: 4 servings
Calories: 388   Calcium: 632 mg.

Edita's Tip: Sardines are a very good source of calcium and there are so many wonderful varieties. I used sardines in tomato sauce for this recipe, but you can also get sardines in mustard, and even in plain water. Don't forget to eat the bones, too.

Salmon Salad

2 cups Romaine salad, torn into chunks
1 cup cherry tomatoes, cut in half
4 green onion, chopped fine
½ cup reduced fat Italian salad dressing
½ cup plain nonfat yogurt
1 can (7-ounces) salmon, drained
¼ teaspoon pepper

Combine all ingredients in a large bowl. Mix well. Serve.

Makes: 2 servings
Calories: 267   Calcium: 372 mg

Tomato & Mozzarella Salad

½ pound skim milk Mozzarella, sliced into 4 thick slices
1 large tomato, sliced into thick slices
½ cup fresh basil leaves, shredded
½ teaspoon salt
¼ teaspoon black pepper
2 tablespoons olive oil

Arrange the cheese and tomato in alternating slices.
Sprinkle with basil, salt and pepper and drizzle with olive
oil. Serve. (Go very easy on the salt or try to omit entirely).

Makes: 2 servings
Calories: 452   Calcium: 844 mg

Broccoli Salad

4 cups broccoli flowerets
1 zucchini, sliced thin
1 green pepper, seeded and sliced into thin slivers
1 red pepper, seeded and sliced into thin slivers
1 cup mushrooms, sliced thin
12 cherry tomatoes, cut into halves
3 green onions, sliced thin
½ cup fat free sour cream
½ cup fat free mayonnaise
½ cup plain, nonfat yogurt
3 cloves garlic, minced
¼ cup skim milk
¼ cup skim milk powder
½ cup blue cheese, crumbled

In a large bowl combine all the ingredients. Toss to coat well. Serve.

Makes: 8 servings
Calories: 85   Calcium: 159 mg

Edita's Tip: Broccoli is a wonderful salad veggie—lots of flavor, crunch and vitamins. Try it!

Fresh Cream of Tomato Soup

1 can (14-ounces) condensed cream of tomato soup
1 can (14-ounces) skim milk
2 tomatoes, chopped
2 spring onions, chopped
1 teaspoon fresh dill, chopped fine
¼ teaspoon black pepper

1. In a medium saucepan, combine all the ingredients and heat. Do not allow to boil. Serve.

Makes: 4 servings
Calories: 86   Calcium: 141 mg

Quick Creamy Asparagus Soup

1 can (14-ounces) condensed cream of asparagus soup
1 can (14-ounces) chicken broth
1 can (14-ounces) skim milk
¼ teaspoon nutmeg

1. In a medium saucepan combine the cream of asparagus soup, broth and skim milk.
2. Heat through. Do not bring to boiling. Serve. Sprinkle each serving with nutmeg.

Makes: 6 servings
Calories: 39   Calcium: 88 mg

Salmon Chowder

1 tablespoon margarine
1 onion, peeled and chopped fine
1 clove garlic, peeled and chopped fine
2 cups chicken broth
1 potato, peeled and diced
1 can (7 ½-ounces) salmon, un-drained, flaked
1 green pepper, seeded and chopped fine
1 red pepper, seeded and chopped fine
¼ teaspoon black pepper
2 cups plain, nonfat yogurt
¼ cup all-purpose flour

1. In a large nonstick saucepan melt the margarine over medium heat. Add the onion and garlic. Cook stirring often until soft, about 2 minutes.
2. Stir in the chicken broth, potatoes. Bring to a boil. Reduce heat and simmer until potatoes are tender.
3. Reduce heat to low and add the corn, salmon, peppers, and black pepper. Simmer. Do not allow the mixture to boil.
4. In a bowl whisk together the yogurt and flour.
5. Gradually add the yogurt mixture to the hot soup stirring constantly until smooth and thickened. Serve.

Makes: 4 servings
Calories: 249   Calcium: 360 mg

Cheddar Cheese Soup

1 can (14-ounces) cream of potato soup
1 can (14-ounces) chicken broth
1 can (14-ounces) skim milk
½ cup low fat cheddar cheese, shredded
¼ teaspoon white pepper

1. Combine all ingredients in a nonstick saucepan.
2. Cook and heat on low heat until cheese melts, stirring often. Do not allow soup to boil. Serve.

Makes: 4 servings
Calories: 89   Calcium: 189 mg

Broccoli Cheddar Soup

1 can (14-ounces) cream of potato soup
1 can (14-ounces) chicken broth
1 can (14-ounces) skim milk
1 package frozen broccoli, chopped
½ cup low fat cheddar cheese, shredded
¼ teaspoon white pepper

1. Combine all ingredients in a nonstick saucepan.
2. Cook and heat on low heat until cheese melts, stirring often. Do not allow soup to boil. Serve.

Makes: 6 servings
Calories: 89   Calcium: 190 mg

Russian Borscht

1 can (16 ounces) seasoned tomatoes, un-drained
2 cans (14-ounces) beef broth
1 onion, peeled and chopped
1 stalk celery, chopped
½ cup parsley, chopped
1 small cabbage, shredded
3 cups spinach, chopped fine
3 tablespoons dill, chopped fine
1 can (14-ounces) beets, sliced
½ cup cider vinegar
½ teaspoon salt
¼ teaspoon pepper
1 teaspoon sugar
1 bay leaf
1 container (8-ounces) plain, nonfat yogurt

1. In a large saucepan combine all the ingredient except for the yogurt.
2. Bring to a boil. Reduce heat. Simmer until the vegetables are tender, about 30 to 40 minutes.
3. Serve garnished with yogurt.

Makes: 6 servings
Calories: 114   Calcium: 183 mg

Italian Cheese Spaghetti Squash

4 cups spaghetti squash, cooked and separated into strands
4 tablespoons Romano cheese, grated
4 tablespoons Parmesan cheese, grated
¼ teaspoon pepper
4 teaspoons parsley, chopped fine

In a large bowl combine all the ingredients. Toss. Serve warm.

Makes 4 servings
Calories: 92   Calcium: 178

Chicken Nuggets

1 pound chicken breasts, skinless, boneless, cut into 1-inch chunks
½ cup low fat Italian dressing
¼ cup skim milk powder
4 cups Total® cereal, crushed fine

Preheat oven to 425°F
1. Mix together the dressing and skim milk powder in a shallow dish.
2. Place the cereal into another shallow dish.
3. Dip the chicken pieces into the dressing mix and then into the cereal making sure each piece is well coated.
4. Place in a single layer in a nonstick baking pan sprayed with cooking spray. Bake 15 minutes or until juices run clear. Serve hot.

Makes: 8 servings
Calories: 116   Calcium: 80 mg approx.

Italian Mozzarella Nuggets

8 ounces part skim Mozzarella cheese, cut into 1-inch
cubes
1 egg
2 tablespoons skim milk
1 cup seasoned breadcrumbs
2 teaspoons garlic powder
2 teaspoons onion powder
2 tablespoons chopped parsley
¼ cup all-purpose flour

Preheat oven to 400°F
1. In a shallow dish combine the egg and milk. In a
   second shallow dish combine the breadcrumbs,
   spices and parsley. In a third dish place the flour.
2. Dip the cheese chunks, first into the flour, then the
   egg, then the breadcrumb mixture coating
   completely with each mixture. Chill 2 hours.
3. Bake on a nonstick cookie sheet sprayed with
   cooking spray until browned and crisp about 5-8
   minutes. Cool slightly.

Makes: 12 servings
Calories: 108   Calcium: 156 mg

Blue Cheese Mushroom Caps

12 large fresh mushrooms
1 bunch scallions or green onions, chopped fine
¼ cup blue cheese, crumbled
1 tablespoon Worcestershire sauce
¼ cup seasoned breadcrumbs
¼ cup Total® cereal, crushed fine

Preheat oven to 350°F
1. Combine the cereal and breadcrumbs in a bowl.
2. Clean mushrooms and remove and chop stems.
3. In a medium nonstick skillet sprayed with cooking spray sauté the scallions and chopped mushroom stems until tender. Add the blue cheese, Worchester sauce and ½ the breadcrumb mixture. Stir until ingredients are combined.
4. Spoon the mixture into the prepared mushroom caps. Arrange on nonstick cookie sheet sprayed with cooking spray. Sprinkle the remaining breadcrumb mixture on top. Bake for 12 to 15 minutes or until hot.

Makes: 12 servings
Calories: 27   Calcium: 22 mg

Night Cap

1 cup skim milk
1 teaspoon sugar
¼ teaspoon cinnamon

Heat all the ingredients together. Serve.

Makes: 1 serving
Calories: 103   Calcium: 309 mg

Mint Lemon Shake

1 cup lemon sherbet
1 cup skim milk
½ cup mint leaves

In a blender combine sherbet and skim milk. Process until smooth. Serve garnished with mint leaves.
Makes: 2 servings
Calories: 150   Calcium: 391 mg

Chocolate Mint Shake

1 cup low fat chocolate mint ice cream
1 cup skim milk
½ cup mint leaves
In a blender combine sherbet and skim milk. Process until smooth. Serve garnished with mint leaves.
Makes: 2 servings
Calories: 168   Calcium: 302 mg

Black & White Shake

1 container (8 ounces) lowfat vanilla yogurt
8 ounces diet cola
Place all ingredients into a blender and process until
smooth. Serve.
Makes: 2 servings.
Calories: 97   Calcium: 199 mg
Edita's Tip: Go easy on this one. It's best saved for an
occasional treat because of the soda.

Green Garden Cocktail

3 kale leaves, washed
3 collard leaves, washed
¼ cup chopped parsley
1 carrot, washed
In a juicer, liquefy all the ingredients. Serve.
Makes 1 serving
Calories: 50   Calcium: 108 mg

Powerhouse Cocktail

4 kale leaves, washed
½ cup fresh broccoli, washed and cut into chunks
½ head of fresh cabbage, cut into chunks
2 carrots, washed, cut into chunks
¼ cup fresh parsley, washed
In a juicer, liquefy all ingredients. Serve
Makes 2 servings
Calories: 143   Calcium: 49 mg

Classic Eggplant Parmesan

1 eggplant, peeled and sliced into ¼ inch rounds
½ pound Mozzarella cheese, part skim
2 tomatoes, sliced thick
¼ cup vegetable oil
½ cup breadcrumbs, Italian seasoned variety
1 egg, slightly beaten
1 cup tomato sauce
¼ teaspoon pepper

Preheat oven to 450°F
1. Place the beaten egg into a shallow dish. Place the
    breadcrumbs and pepper into a shallow dish. Dip
    the eggplant slices, first into the egg and then into
    the breadcrumbs, coating both sides.
2. In a nonstick saucepan heat the oil and sauté the
    breaded eggplant. Remove and drain on paper
    towels.
3. In a nonstick casserole layer first the eggplant, then
    the tomatoes, then the tomato sauce and finish with
    a layer of the cheese. Bake for 15 to 20 minutes
    until cheese is golden and bubbly. Serve hot.

Makes: 6 servings
Calories: 275   Calcium: 304 mg

Spinach Casserole

1 package (10-ounces) frozen spinach, cooked, drained and chopped
1 onion, peeled and chopped
2 tomatoes, sliced
1 tub (16-ounces) low fat cottage cheese
¼ cup Parmesan cheese, grated
¼ cup Romano cheese, grated
½ teaspoon basil
½ teaspoon oregano
¼ teaspoon black pepper

Preheat oven to 350ºF
1. Place cottage cheese, onion and spices into a blender or food processor. Process until smooth.
2. Layer alternating layers of spinach, cheese mixture and tomatoes in a nonstick casserole. Top with the two cheeses. Bake, uncovered for 25 to 30 minutes. Serve hot.

Makes: 6 servings
Calories: 116   Calcium: 205 mg

Hearty Stuffed Tomatoes

6 large tomatoes
1 package (10-ounces) frozen spinach, thawed, drained, chopped
8 ounces Ricotta cheese, part skim
2 ½ cups Fontina cheese, part skim, grated
¾ cup Parmesan cheese, grated
¼ teaspoon black pepper
½ cup parsley, chopped fine
½ teaspoon anchovy paste
2 cloves garlic, peeled and minced

Preheat oven to 400°F
1. Peel tomatoes by dipping them into boiling water for a minute, letting them cook and pulling off the skin. Cut the top off each tomato and scoop out the seeds.
2. In a bowl, mix together the spinach and cheeses. Add the remaining ingredients. Combine well.
3. Stuff each tomato with the cheese mixture. Bake for 5-10 minutes until heated through and the cheeses are melted. Serve hot.

Makes: 12 servings
Calories: 157   Calcium: 278 mg

Broccoli Stir-Fry

1 pound broccoli, cut into flowerets
1 tablespoon vegetable oil
½ teaspoon soy sauce, reduced sodium
1 teaspoon rice wine
¼ teaspoon sugar
3 tablespoons chicken broth
¼ cup water

1. Heat oil in a nonstick skillet or wok over high heat. Add the broccoli and stir-fry for 1 minute.
2. Add the remaining ingredients.
3. Reduce heat and continue to cook until the water is evaporated. Serve hot.

Makes: 2 servings
Calories: 136   Calcium: 111 mg

Garlicky Greens Dinner

1 onion, peeled and chopped fine
6 cloves garlic, peeled and minced
1 pound kale, washed and chopped
1 pound collard greens, washed and chopped
½ cup chicken broth
2 tablespoons lemon juice
¼ teaspoon lemon zest
¼ teaspoon black pepper

1. Spray a large saucepan with cooking spray and heat over medium heat. Sauté the onion and garlic 2-3 minutes until tender.
2. Add the greens and broth. Heat to boiling. Reduce heat, cover and simmer for 5 minutes.
3. Add the lemon and pepper. Toss. Serve hot.

Makes: 4 servings
Calories: 115   Calcium: 334 mg

Quick & Easy Salmon Casserole

2 cups peas, cooked and drained
1 can (14-ounces) cream of chicken soup
1 cup plain nonfat yogurt
2 cans (7-ounces each) canned salmon, drained, with bones
1 onion, peeled and chopped fine

Preheat oven to 350°F
1. In a large bowl combine all the ingredients. Toss to combine.
2. Put into a nonstick casserole sprayed with cooking spray. Bake uncovered for 30 minutes or until heated through. Serve hot.

Makes: 6 servings
Calories: 197   Calcium: 244 mg

Edita's Tip: Serve this wonderful dish with a large green salad or some crisp steamed broccoli, or my personal favorite, a juicy tomato sliced thick and topped with chopped green onion and a little crumbled blue cheese.

Veal Parmesan

4 veal cutlets, ¼ inch thick
½ cup breadcrumbs, seasoned
4 tablespoons Parmesan cheese, grated
1 egg
1 tablespoon skim milk
1 ½ cups spaghetti sauce
½ cup part skim Mozzarella cheese, shredded
¼ teaspoon oregano
¼ teaspoon black pepper

Preheat oven to 375°F
1. Place veal cutlets between 2 sheets of waxed paper and pound until half as thin.
2. In a shallow dish mix together the breadcrumbs, Parmesan cheese. In another shallow dish mix together the egg and milk.
3. Dip each cutlet first into the egg mixture and then into the breadcrumb mixture. Coating well on both sides.
4. Heat a large skillet sprayed with cooking spray over medium heat. Brown the veal on both sides.
5. Arrange veal in a single layer in a nonstick casserole. Pour sauce over the veal. Sprinkle with the Mozzarella and oregano and pepper. Bake 30 minutes or until bubbly. Serve hot.

Makes: 4 servings
Calories: 564   Calcium: 259 mg

Swiss Baked Chicken

6 chicken breasts, skinless and boneless
1 ½ cups reduced fat Swiss cheese, shredded
1 can (10 ¾ ounces) condensed cream of chicken soup
½ cup skim milk
¼ teaspoon pepper

Preheat oven to 350°F
1. Spray a large baking dish with cooking spray.
2. Place chicken breasts in a single layer. Sprinkle with cheese.
3. In a small bowl combine the soup, milk and pepper.
4. Pour the mixture over the chicken and cheese.
5. Bake covered for 1 hour or until chicken is tender. Serve hot.

Makes: 6 servings
Calories: 384   Calcium: 337 mg

Edita's Tip: Try making this with some sliced mushrooms and mushroom soup—delicious!

Salmon Burgers

1 can (16-ounces) salmon, with liquid
1 onion, peeled and grated
½ cup Total® cereal, crushed fine
2 eggs
1 teaspoon dry mustard
½ cup breadcrumbs, seasoned

1. In a medium bowl combine all the ingredients. Mash with a fork until well combined. Shape into patties.
2. Spray a nonfat skillet with cooking spray and heat over medium heat. Brown patties on both sides. Drain on paper towels. Serve warm.

Makes: 4 servings
Calories: 289   Calcium: 281 mg approx

Classic Meatloaf

2 pounds lean ground beef
2 eggs
1 cup skim milk powder
1 onion, peeled and grated
½ cup bread crumbs, seasoned
½ teaspoon garlic powder
¼ teaspoon black pepper

Preheat oven to 350°F
1. In a bowl, mix all ingredients together.
2. Spray a loaf pan with cooking spray. Place the beef mixture into the loaf pan and bake, covered for 1 ½ hours. Serve hot.

Makes: 8 servings
Calories: 348   Calcium: 118 mg

Edita's Tip: This is wonderful served cold and wrapped in big leaves of Romaine lettuce with a little of your favorite mustard.

Meatless Chili

1 ½ cups carrot, peeled and sliced thin
2 onions, peeled and chopped fine
1 green pepper, seeded and chopped fine
1 red pepper, seeded and chopped fine
1 ½ cups celery, sliced fine
1 cup skim milk powder
1 can (15-ounces) stewed tomatoes
1 can (15-ounces) tomato sauce
1 can (6-ounces) tomato paste
1 can (6-ounces) tomato juice
½ cup salsa
juice of 1 lemon
2 cans (15-ounces) kidney beans, with liquid
1 can (15-ounces) chickpeas
3 cloves garlic, peeled and chopped fine
3 tablespoons chili powder
1 ½ teaspoons basil
½ teaspoon black pepper
1 teaspoon pepper sauce

1. Combine all ingredients in a large, nonstick saucepan.
2. Simmer, covered on low-medium heat, until tender stirring occasionally about 20-minutes. Do not overcook. Serve hot.

Makes: 12 servings
Calories: 193   Calcium: 194 mg

Cheese Omelet

4 eggs
4 tablespoons skim milk
½ cup low fat Cheddar cheese, shredded
¼ teaspoon pepper
½ teaspoon parsley, chopped fine

1. In a bowl mix the eggs, milk, pepper and parsley.
2. Spray a nonstick omelet pan or skillet with sloping sides, with cooking spray and place over medium heat.
3. Pour the egg mixture into the pan and cook, drawing the edges of the mixture away from the sides of the pan letting the uncooked portion flow underneath. Cook until the mixture is no longer runny.
4. Sprinkle the top with cheese. Fold over using a spatula. Slide onto plate and serve hot.

Makes: 2 servings
Calories: 191   Calcium: 200 mg

Edita's Tip: Try different cheeses with this omelet. You can also add a handful of leftover cooked vegetables, fresh mushrooms or fresh tomatoes. Be imaginative. Enjoy!

Cheese & Vegetable Frittata

2 tablespoons chicken stock
1 cup zucchini, sliced thin
2 tomatoes, seeded, peeled and chopped fine
1 green pepper, seeded and sliced into strips
1 onion, peeled and sliced thin, separated into rings
½ teaspoon basil
½ teaspoon oregano
8 eggs
½ cup skim milk
¼ teaspoon pepper
1 cup part skim Mozzarella cheese, shredded

Preheat oven to 350°F.
1. In an oven proof, nonstick skillet sauté the zucchini, tomato, pepper, and onion in the chicken stock until the vegetables are tender. Add the spices. Transfer the vegetables to a bowl.
2. Combine the eggs and milk in a bowl.
3. Heat the oven proof skillet and spray with cooking spray. Pour in the eggs. Cook drawing the egg mixture in at the edges toward the center using a spatula so the liquid flows to the bottom.
4. While the top is still moist sprinkle with the vegetable mixture and cheese. Bake 5 minutes or until cheese melts and top is golden. Slide onto a serving plate and serve.

Makes: 4 servings
Calories: 259   Calcium: 311 mg

Hamburger Casserole

2 pounds lean ground beef
1 cup reduced fat cottage cheese
½ cup reduced fat sour cream,
¼ cup skim milk powder
½ cup tomato paste
½ teaspoon garlic powder
¼ teaspoon black pepper
6 green onion, chopped fine
1 cup low fat cheddar cheese, shredded

Preheat broiler
1. Brown the beef in a nonstick ovenproof skillet sprayed with cooking spray, stirring often until browned and crumbled and cooked through.
2. Mix in the cottage cheese, sour cream, tomato paste, skim milk powder, garlic powder, pepper and green onion. Top with the cheddar cheese.
3. Place under the broiler for 5 minutes or until cheese melts.

Makes: 6 servings
Calories: 444   Calcium: 138 mg

Seafood Florentine

2 lb fish fillets
1 onion, peeled and sliced thin
1 teaspoon olive oil
1 package (10-ounces) frozen spinach, thawed, drained, chopped
1 tablespoon lemon juice
1 teaspoon soy sauce, low sodium
¼ teaspoon paprika
¼ teaspoon pepper

Preheat oven to 350°F
1. In a nonstick skillet sprayed with cooking spray heat the olive oil and cook the onion until soft.
2. Add the spinach. Cook until heated through.
3. Add the lemon juice, soy sauce, paprika and pepper.
4. Place the spinach mixture in the bottom of a nonstick baking dish sprayed with cooking. Arrange the fish fillets on top.
5. Bake for 30 minutes or until fish flakes.

Makes: 4 servings
Calories: 226   Calcium: 122 mg

Hearty Irish Stew

2 pounds sirloin, trimmed of fat and cut into chunks
1 can (14-ounces) cream of mushroom soup
1 envelope onion soup mix
½ cup skim milk powder
½ teaspoon black pepper
1 cup beef broth
2 potatoes, peeled and cut into chunks
4 carrots, peeled and cut into chunks
2 onions, peeled and cut into chunks

Preheat oven to 350°F
1. Spray a casserole with cooking spray.
2. Mix together the meat, mushroom soup, onion soup, pepper and chicken broth and bake covered for 45 minutes.
3. Add the vegetables and cover and continue to bake until vegetables are tender and the stew is thick and hot. Serve hot.

Makes: 6 servings
Calories: 474   Calcium: 184 mg

Edita's Tip: This is a wonderful winter dish and it smells great coming from the oven. It's my absolutely favorite stew recipe.

Vegetable Lasagna

1 onion, peeled and chopped
2 cloves garlic, peeled and minced
2 carrots, peeled and diced
1 stalk celery, peeled and diced
2 cups mushrooms, diced
1 can (16-ounces) seasoned tomatoes
1 can (8-ounces) tomato sauce
1 package (10-ounces) frozen spinach, thawed, chopped
3 cups broccoli florets
1 teaspoon each oregano and basil
½ teaspoon black pepper
9 lasagna noodles, cooked and drained
1 cup reduced fat cottage cheese
2 cups low fat Mozzarella cheese, shredded
½ cup Parmesan, grated
½ cup skim milk powder

Preheat oven to 350ºF
In a nonstick skillet sprayed with cooking spray, cook the onion and garlic until soft, about 2 minutes. Add the celery, mushrooms, tomatoes, tomato sauce, spinach, broccoli and spices. Cook until the vegetables uncovered 10-15 minutes. Spray a large nonstick baking pan with cooking spray and layer the noodles, vegetable mixture, cottage cheese and Mozzarella, repeating layers. Top with noodle layer and sprinkle with remaining Mozzarella and Parmesan. Bake 40 to 45 minutes until bubbly.

Makes: 8 servings
Calories: 533   Calcium: 403 mg

Baked Leeks With Cheese Supper

8 leeks, washed, sliced into ¼ inch rounds, white part only
2 tablespoons reduced fat margarine
2 tablespoons dry white wine
¾ cup reduced fat Muenster cheese, grated
¼ teaspoon black pepper

Preheat oven to 350°F
1. In a small nonstick casserole sprayed with cooking spray combine the leeks, margarine, wine and pepper. Toss gently until well combined.
2. Bake for 30 minutes or until leeks are tender.
3. Sprinkle with cheese and place under broiler until cheese bubbles. Serve hot.

Makes: 4 servings
Calories: 217   Calcium: 259 mg

Edita's Tip: I love leeks. Here's one of my favorite quick soups—and I've even served it at a dinner party and got raves. Nobody guessed how easy it was. Chop and rinse about 4 leeks—just the white part. In a small nonstick saucepan empty your basic can of chicken stock and simmer the leeks in the stock for about 5 minutes. Don't over cook them. Mix in your basic can of cream of potato soup and a couple of teaspoons of nonfat powdered skim milk. Heat through. Serve. How easy was that?

Fresh Vegetable Casserole

4 garlic cloves, minced
2 tablespoons olive oil
2 tomatoes, chopped
½ pound green beans, cut into small chunks
½ pound peas, fresh or frozen
½ cup feta cheese, crumbled
1 teaspoon oregano
¼ teaspoon pepper

1. In a large, nonstick skillet sprayed with cooking spray, sauté the garlic in the olive oil until softened, about 2 minutes.
2. Add the tomatoes, beans, and peas. Cover and simmer until vegetables are tender, about 5 to 7 minutes.
3. Add the cheese and spices. Heat until cheese is melted. Serve warm.

Makes: 4 servings
Calories: 187   Calcium: 138 mg

Edita's Tip: The beauty of this recipe is you can use whatever veggies you happen to have in the fridge. It's a great way to use up leftovers, or even those few frozen veggies that don't quite make up a whole side dish on their own.

Lean Creamed Spinach Dinner

2 packages (10-ounces) frozen spinach, cooked and drained
1 onion, peeled and chopped fine
2 cloves garlic, peeled and chopped fine
1 tablespoon all-purpose flour
¾ cup skim milk
¼ cup powdered skim milk
¼ cup Parmesan cheese, grated
¼ teaspoon nutmeg
¼ teaspoon black pepper

1. Keep cooked spinach hot.
2. In a nonstick saucepan sprayed with cooking spray, sauté the onion and garlic until soft.
3. Stir in the flour. Cook for 1 minute, stirring constantly.
4. Gradually add the liquid milk, stirring constantly until the mixture thickens.
5. Stir in the powdered skim milk, spices and cheese. Continue cooking until cheese melts.
6. Pour sauce over hot spinach.

Makes: 8 servings
Calories: 47   Calcium: 146 mg

Edita's Tip: Serve this with your favorite meat or try it with the Salmon Burgers. It's wonderful over spaghetti squash, too!

Russian Dressing

1 cup mayonnaise, reduced fat
1 cup cottage cheese, low fat
2 tablespoons skim milk
1 tablespoon lemon juice
1/3 cup tomato juice
1 onion, peeled and chopped fine
¼ cup parsley, chopped fine
½ teaspoon hot sauce

Place all ingredients in a blender or food processor. Process until smooth. Store covered in fridge.

Makes: 12 servings
Calories: 72   Calcium: 19 mg

Edita's Tip: This dressing is great on a small tin of tuna for lunch and it works equally well as a dip for assorted veggies as a TV snack.

Thousand Island Dressing

1 cup, plain, nonfat yogurt
3 tablespoons, reduced fat mayonnaise
2 tablespoons pickle relish
1 tablespoon skim milk
1 tablespoon onion, peeled and chopped fine
1 tablespoon green pepper, seeded and chopped fine
1 tablespoon red pepper, seeded and chopped fine
garlic powder to taste
¼ teaspoon black pepper to taste

Combine all ingredients in a small bowl. Cover. Chill for at least 2 hours.

Makes 12 servings
Calories: 25   Calcium: 40 mg

Lemon Tofu Dressing

⅔ cup tofu, drained
3 tablespoons lemon juice
3 tablespoons olive oil
2 teaspoons low-sodium soy sauce
¼ teaspoon pepper to taste

Put all ingredients into a blender or food processor. Process until smooth.

Makes: 1 cup   Serving size: ¼ cup
Calories: 125   Calcium: 45 mg

Spicy Buttermilk Dressing

1 cup buttermilk
1 tablespoon Dijon-style mustard
1 onion, peeled and minced fine
2 teaspoons parsley, chopped
½ teaspoon dill, fresh or dried
¼ teaspoon black pepper to taste

Combine all ingredients in a jar. Shake to mix. Store in fridge tightly covered.

Makes: 4 servings
Calories: 38   Calcium: 82 mg

Peppery Yogurt Dressing

½ cup plain, nonfat yogurt
2 tablespoons lemon juice
generous dash of hot sauce or Tabasco

Place all ingredients into a covered jar. Shake well. Store in fridge tightly covered.

Makes: 4 servings
Calories: 18   Calcium: 57 mg

Chunky Blue Cheese Dressing

½ cup blue cheese, crumbled
1 cup yogurt, plain, nonfat
1 clove garlic, peeled and mashed fine
dry mustard to taste
¼ teaspoon pepper to taste

Place all ingredients in a covered jar. Shake well. Store in fridge tightly covered.

Makes: 6 servings
Calories: 61   Calcium: 74 mg

Parsley Herb Dressing

½ cup fresh parsley, chopped fine
1 cup cottage cheese, low fat
1 teaspoon Dijon-type mustard
1 teaspoon lemon juice
¼ teaspoon black pepper

Place all ingredients in a blender or food processor. Process until smooth.

Makes: 12 servings
Calories: 14   Calcium: 12 mg

Buttermilk Dressing

1 cup buttermilk
1 tablespoon Dijon-type mustard
1 onion, peeled and chopped fine
2 teaspoons parsley, chopped fine
½ teaspoon dill
¼ teaspoon black pepper

Combine all ingredients in a jar with a lid. Shake to combine. Store in fridge tightly covered.

Makes; 12 servings
Calories: 13   Calcium: 28 mg

Parmesan Yogurt Dressing

1 container (8-ounces) plain, nonfat yogurt
½ cup green onions, chopped fine
3 tablespoons parmesan cheese, grated
½ teaspoon salt
¼ teaspoon pepper
½ teaspoon dill

Place all ingredients in blender or food processor. Process until smooth. Store in fridge.

Makes: 8 servings
Calories: 27   Calcium: 89 mg

Caesar Dressing

1 container (8-ounces) plain, nonfat yogurt
1 cup mayonnaise, reduced fat
1 teaspoon lemon juice
2 teaspoons garlic, peeled and chopped fine
2 tablespoons parmesan cheese, grated
½ teaspoon dry mustard
1 teaspoon salt
½ teaspoon pepper

Place all ingredients in a blender or food processor. Process until smooth.

Makes: 12 servings
Calories: 69   Calcium: 52

Edita's Tip: Try putting your dressings in a little side dish. Dip the ends of your fork in the dressing and then spear some salad. You'll get all the dressing taste, with many fewer calories. This is a good eating habit to get into, especially when eating out when you are not really sure of all the ingredients in the salad dressings available.

Garden Spinach Dip

2 cups plain, nonfat yogurt
1 package (10-oz) frozen spinach, thawed, chopped, drained
⅓ cup onion, peeled and chopped fine
2 tablespoons reduced fat mayonnaise
1 package instant vegetable soup mix

In a medium bowl combine yogurt all ingredients. Mix well. Serve immediately or cover and chill up to 3-hours.

Makes 24 servings
Calories: 18   Calcium: 52

Mexican Chili Dip

⅔ cup plain, nonfat yogurt
⅓ cup reduced fat mayonnaise
¼ cup green pepper, seeded and chopped fine
¼ cup red pepper, seeded and chopped fine
¼ cup chili sauce
2 tablespoons green onion, chopped fine
1 tablespoon horseradish

Combine all ingredients. Cover. Chill.

Makes 12 servings
Calories: 28   Calcium: 28 mg

Cheese Cake Pie

1 prepared graham cracker crust
2 cups low fat cottage cheese
2 tablespoons Butter Buds®
4 egg whites
½ cup sugar
½ cup skim milk
¼ cup skim milk powder
¼ cup all-purpose flour
1 tablespoon grated lemon peel
2 tablespoons lemon juice

Preheat oven to 300°F
1. In a blender or food processor combine the all the ingredients, one at a time, blending well after each addition.
2. Pour the mixture into the prepared crust. Bake for 90 minutes until firm. Cool.

Makes: 8 servings
Calories: 286   Calcium: 110 mg

Edita's Tip: I like to spoon some fresh fruit on this dessert. Try berries, or tropical fruits, or just garnish with a few slices of fresh lemon. Enjoy.

Creamy Cheesecake Cookies

½ cup liquid Butter Buds®
1 cup sugar
1 egg, lightly beaten
1 package (3-ounces) low fat cream cheese
2 tablespoons plain, nonfat yogurt
1 teaspoon vanilla
2 cups all-purpose flour
⅛ teaspoon baking soda
½ teaspoon baking powder

Preheat oven to 350° F
1. In a mixing bowl, cream together the Butter Buds, sugar and egg.
2. Add the cheese and the yogurt. Blend again until creamy.
3. Add the remaining ingredients. Beat until smooth.
4. Form the dough into a ball and chill in fridge for 2 hours.
5. Remove from fridge and roll out thin and cut into shapes, using the bottom of glass or your favorite cookie shapes.
6. Bake for 12 minutes or until golden brown. Cool on wire rack.

Makes: 36 cookies
Calories: 60

Serving size: 1 cookie
Calcium: 10 mg

Banana Cream Pie

1 prepared graham cracker pie crust
1 package instant vanilla pudding mix
1 cup skim milk
1 cup low fat vanilla yogurt
2 bananas, peeled and sliced thin

1. Prepare pudding according to package directions using both the yogurt and skim milk.
2. Arrange the banana sliced on the bottom of the prepared piecrust reserving a few slices for a garnish. Pour the pudding on top.
3. Chill until set.
4. Top with remaining banana slices. Serve.

Makes: 8 servings
Calories: 228   Calcium: 113 mg

Strawberry Cream Pie

1 prepared graham cracker pie crust
1 package instant strawberry pudding mix
1 cup skim milk
1 cup low fat strawberry yogurt
2 cups strawberries, hulled and sliced

1. Prepare pudding according to package directions using both the yogurt and skim milk.
2. Arrange the strawberry slices on the bottom of the prepared piecrust reserving a few slices for a garnish. Pour the pudding on top.
3. Chill until set.
4. Top with remaining strawberry slices. Serve.

Makes: 8 servings
Calories: 216   Calcium: 107 mg

Pink & Blush Trifle

½ cup jellied cranberry sauce
3 tablespoons water
1 package instant vanilla pudding mix
1 cup skim milk
1 cup low fat vanilla yogurt
12 lady fingers, split
1 ½ cups peach slices, fresh or frozen, washed and drained
1 ½ cups fresh strawberries, hulled and sliced

1. In a small saucepan heat the cranberry sauce and water until cranberry sauce is melted. Beat with a wire whisk until smooth. Set aside until cool.
2. Prepare pudding mixture according to package directions using both the skim milk and yogurt.
3. In a straight-edged serving bowl, arrange enough lady fingers to cover bottom and sides of the dish.
4. Layer half the peaches, strawberries, pudding, and lady fingers in the bowl. Pour a little of the cranberry mixture over the first layer. Repeat the layers with the remaining ingredients.
5. Cover. Chill for 4 hours. Serve.

Makes: 12 servings
Calories: 128   Calcium: 79 mg

Apple Cinnamon Tart

1 ½ cups quick-cooking oats
1 tablespoon + ½ teaspoon cinnamon
¾ cup frozen apple juice concentrate, thawed
2 large apples, cored and sliced thin
1 teaspoon lemon juice
⅓ cup cold water
1 envelope unflavored gelatin
2 cups plain nonfat yogurt
¼ cup honey
½ teaspoon almond extract

Preheat oven to 350°F
1. In a small bowl combine the oats and 1 tablespoon cinnamon. Toss with ¼ cup of the apple juice concentrate. Press onto the bottom and side of a nonstick 9-inch pie plate sprayed with cooking spray. Bake 5 minutes. Cool on wire rack.
2. In a medium bowl toss apple slices with lemon juice. Arrange in a layer on the cooled crust.
3. In a small nonstick saucepan combine cold water and remaining ½ cup of the apple juice concentrate. Sprinkle the gelatin over water mixture. Let stand 3 minutes to soften. Cook over medium heat stirring until gelatin is dissolved. Remove from heat. Add yogurt, honey, ½ teaspoon of cinnamon and the almond extract. Mix well. Pour over the apples in the crust. Chill overnight. Serve

Makes: 8 servings
Calories: 197   Calcium: 138 mg

Frosty Fruit Yogurt Pie

1 graham cracker prepared piecrust
1 pint reduced fat frozen strawberry yogurt, slightly softened
1 pint fresh strawberries, hulled and sliced thin

Fill the piecrust with the yogurt. Arrange strawberry slices on top. Return to freezer for a few minutes. Serve cold

Makes: 8 servings
Calories:205   Calcium: 58 mg

Edita's Tip: Non fat yogurt, plain or frozen is a wonderful treat. Try it lots of different ways. In chilled pies. Topped with fruit. As the frosty part of a banana split. As part of a shake or smoothie. Your body will thank you.

Fruity Yogurt Cup

4 cups fresh fruit or berries, chopped
2 cups fat free vanilla yogurt

Alternate layers of fresh fruit and yogurt in tall parfait glasses. Serve.

Makes: 8 servings
Calories: 84   Calcium: 114 mg

Yogurt Pudding

1 package fruit-flavored jello mix
1 cup nonfat fruit yogurt

Prepare jello according to package directions. Chill until it begins to set. Stir in the yogurt. Mix well. Chill until set. Serve cold.

Makes: 4 servings
Calories: 62   Calcium: 86 mg

Quick Coffee Cake

1 ½ cups all-purpose flour
1 cup granulated sugar
2 teaspoons baking powder
½ teaspoon baking soda
1 cup plain nonfat yogurt
2 eggs

Preheat oven to 350°F
1. In a large bowl mix together the flour, sugar, baking powder and baking soda.
2. In another bowl combine the eggs and the yogurt. Beat thoroughly.
3. Add the dry ingredients to the yogurt mixture. Beat until smooth.
4. Pour into a 9 x 9-inch nonstick baking pan sprayed with cooking spray. Bake for 20 minutes. Serve warm.

Makes: 8 servings
Calories: 215   Calcium: 133 mg

New York Cheesecake

1 prepared graham cracker piecrust
3 package (8-ounces each) fat free cream cheese, softened
¾ cup sugar
2 eggs
2 tablespoons cornstarch
1 teaspoon vanilla
½ cup reduced fat sour cream
½ cup plain nonfat yogurt

Preheat oven to 325°F
1. Beat together in a large bowl the cheese and sugar until light and fluffy.
2. Beat in eggs, vanilla and cornstarch.
3. Add the sour cream and yogurt. Mix well.
4. Pour into the prepared piecrust. Bake 45 minutes until firm. Serve chilled.

Makes: 12 servings
Calories: 320   Calcium: 90 mg

Macaroons

4 egg whites
⅛ teaspoon cream of tartar
¼ teaspoon salt
1 cup sugar
¼ cup skim milk powder
1 cup canned sweetened coconut

Preheat oven to 300°F
1. In a medium bowl beat together the egg whites, cream of tartar and salt until soft peaks form.
2. Beat in the sugar until peaks stiffen. Fold in coconut.
3. Drop by teaspoonfuls on a nonstick cookie sheet sprayed with cooking spray. Bake until slightly browned about 20 minutes. Cool.

Makes: 24 servings
Calories: 51   Calcium: 17 mg

Chewy Chocolate Brownies

1 cup all-purpose flour
1 cup sugar
¼ cup unsweetened cocoa
6 tablespoons reduced fat margarine, melted
¼ cup skim milk
¼ cup skim milk powder
1 egg
2 egg whites
1 teaspoon vanilla extract
¼ cup honey

Preheat oven to 350°F
1. In a large bowl mix together all the ingredients.
2. Pour the mixture into a nonstick 8 by 8-inch baking pan sprayed with cooking spray. Bake for 30 minutes or until brownies spring back when touched lightly. Cool.

Makes: 24 servings
Calories: 88   Calcium: 23 mg

Part Five

The Resources Part

National Institutes of Health
Dietary Reference Intakes

CATEGORY	RDA/AIPER DAY
Infants from birth to 6 months	210 mg
Infants from 7 months to 12 months	270 mg
Children from 1 to 3 years	500 mg
Children from 4 to 8 years	800 mg
Males	
9 to 13 years	1300 mg
14 to 18 years	1300 mg
19 to 30 years	1000 mg
31 to 50 years	1000 mg
51 to 70 years	1200 mg
Over 70 years	1200 mg
Females	
9 to 13 years	1300 mg
14 to 18 years	1300 mg
19 to 30 years	1000 mg
31 to 50 years	1000 mg
50 to 70 years	1200 mg
Over 70 years	1200 mg
Pregnancy	
Up to 18 years	1300 mg
19 to 30 years	1000 mg
31 to 50 years	1000 mg
Lactation	
Up to 18 years	1300 mg
19 to 30 years	1000 mg
31 to 50 years	1000 mg

Calcium Diet Super Foods—Dairy Group

FOOD	MG
Yogurt, plain, nonfat, 1 cup	452
Yogurt, plain, low fat, 1 cup	415
Yogurt, fruit-flavored, low fat, 1 cup	314
Milk, skim, 1 cup	302
Milk, 1% low fat, 1 cup	300
Milk, 2% low fat, 1 cup	297
Milk, whole, 1 cup	291
Buttermilk, 1 cup	285
Milk, chocolate, 2% low fat, 1 cup	284
Milk, chocolate, whole, 1 cup	280
Cheese, Swiss, 1 ounce	272
Cheese, Cheddar, 1 ounce	204
Cheese, Mozzarella, part skim, 1 ounce	183
Cheese, American, 1 ounce	174
Ice Milk, soft serve, ½ cup	137
Ice Cream, soft serve, ½ cup	118
Yogurt, frozen, plain, ½ cup	89
Ice cream, 10% fat, ½ cup	88
Cottage cheese, 2% low fat, ½ cup	77

Calcium Super Foods—Protein Group

FOOD	MG
Tofu, ½ cup with calcium sulphate	434
Sardines, canned with bones	324
Salmon, canned with bones	203
Tofu, ½ cup without calcium sulphate	130
Perch, baked, 3 ounces	117
Almonds, ¼ cup	94
Brazil nuts, ¼ cup	62
Beans, great northern, boiled, ½ cup	61
Shrimp, cooked, 3-ounces	33
Egg, hard-cooked, 1 large	28
Peanuts, ¼ cup	21
Pork chop, 3 ounces	13
Peanut butter, 2 tablespoons	10

Calcium Super Foods—Fruit & Veggie Group

FOOD	MG
Spinach, fresh, cooked, ½ cup	122
Turnip greens, fresh, cooked, ½ cup	99
Kale, frozen, cooked, ½ cup	90
Broccoli, fresh, cooked, ½ cup	89
Okra, fresh, cooked, ½ cup	88
Beet greens, fresh, cooked, ½ cup	82
Bokchoy, fresh cooked, ½ cup	79
Mustard greens, frozen, cooked, ½ cup	75
Collards, fresh, cooked, ½ cup	74
Dandelion greens, fresh, cooked, ½ cup	73
Orange, medium	52
Broccoli, frozen, cooked, ½ cup	47
Beans, green, frozen, cooked, ½ cup	31
Potatoes, mashed, ½ cup	28
Summer squash, fresh, cooked, ½ cup	24
Pear, medium, one	19
Peas, green, frozen, cooked, ½ cup	19
Carrots, one medium, raw	19
Raisins, seedless, ¼ cup	18
Iceberg lettuce, 1/8 head	17

Calcium Super Foods—Grain Group

FOOD	MG
Waffle, 7-inches diameter	179
Pancakes, 4-inches diameter, 2	72
Hamburger roll	54
Baking powder biscuit	47
Corn tortilla	42
White bread, one slice	32
Bagel	29
Hard roll	24
Whole wheat bread, one slice	20
Rice, ½ cup	11
Oatmeal, ½ cup	10

Your Personal Calcium Counter

<u>Food</u>   <u>Calcium in mg</u>

Bread
 Black, 1 slice   21.8
 Egg, chalah, 1 slice   27.6
 Italian, 1 slice   16.0
 Pita, 1 small   49.2
 Pumpernickel, 1 slice   21.8
 Raisin, 1 slice   27.3
 Rye, 1 slice   19.5
 Sourdough, 1 slice   22.5
 White, 1 slice   31.2
 Whole wheat, 1 slice   25.7
 Breadsticks, 1   8.2
 Bread stuffing, 1 cup   145.9
 Biscuits, from mix, 1   19.8
Muffins
 Bran, 1   116.4
 English, 1   93.8
Bagels
 Plain, 1   23.1
Cake
 Angel food, 1 slice   41.7
 Carrot, 1 slice   58.9
 Cheesecake, 1 slice   69.3
 Fruitcake, 1 slice   97.9
 Gingerbread, 1 slice   55.9
 Jelly roll, 1 slice   14.7
 Pound cake, 1 slice   55.0
Pies
 Apple, 1 slice   10.8
 Banana cream, 1 slice   85.4
 Custard, 1 slice   120.9
 Mince, 1 slice   38.5
Cereals
 Bran, 1 cup   69

Cheerios, 1 cup	48
Total, 1 cup	250
Wheaties, 1 cup	43
Cheese	
Blue, 1 ounce	149.6
Brick, 1 ounce	162.0
Brie, 1 ounce	52.2
Camembert, 1 ounce	109.9
Cheddar, 1 ounce	204.5
Colby, 1 ounce	165.0
Cottage cheese, 4 oz	67.8
Cottage cheese, low fat, 4 oz	77.4
Edam, 1 ounce	207.2
Feta, 1 ounce	139.6
Monterey, 1 ounce	211.6
Mozzarella, part skim, 1 ounce	183.1
Parmesan, grated, 1 ounce	335.5
Ricotta, part skim, 1 ounce	337.3
Swiss, 1 ounce	213.0
American processed, 1 ounce	174.0
Fruit	
Apricots, 3 raw	15
Avocado, 1	21
Dried figs, ½ cup	269
Kiwi fruit, 1	20
Cantaloupe, ½	28
Orange, 1	52
Raisins, 1 cup	71
Strawberries, 1 cup	21
Watermelon, 1 slice	38
Legumes	
Baked beans, ½ cup	77.9
Chickpeas, ½ cup	59.9
Pinto beans, ½ cup	39.9
Red kidney beans, ½ cup	34.6
White beans, ½ cup	45.1
Dairy	
Cream, half & half, 1 tbsp	15.7
Cream, whipping, 1 tbsp	3

Sour cream, 1 tbsp	14
Milk, whole, 1 cup	290.4
Milk, low fat, 1 cup	296.7
Milk, skim, 1 cup	316.3
Buttermilk, 1 cup	285.2
Chocolate milk, 1 cup	280.2
Ice cream, 1 cup	175.7
Ice milk, 1 cup	176.1
Yogurt, plain, 4 oz	136.9
Yogurt, plain, low fat, 4 oz	207.1
Yogurt, fruit, low fat, 4 oz	172.3

Seafood

Mackerel, canned, 3 oz	263.1
Oysters, raw, 3 oz	79.9
Salmon, broiled, 3 oz	132.9
Salmon, canned 3 oz	190.7
Sardines, canned in oil, 3 oz	371.4

Vegetables

Beans, lima, ½ cup	27
Beans, snap, ½ cup	21
Beet greens, cooked, ½ cup	82
Broccoli, cooked, ½ cup	89
Bok-choy, ½ cup	79
Chard, swiss, ½ cup	51
Collards, ½ cup	109
Kale, ½ cup	47
Okra, ½ cup	88
Spinach, ½ cup	122

Good Sources of Calcium
From the Guidelines on Overweight and Obesity
National Heart, Lung and Blood Institute

Source	Calcium (milligrams)
Milk (1 cup)	
Whole	300
2% reduced-fat	300
1% reduced-fat	300
Fat Free*	300
Yogurt* (1 cup)	
Plain, low fat	415
Flavored, low fat	315
Plain, fat free	315
Cheese (1 ounce)	
Reduced fat Cheddar*	120
American	175
Swiss Cheese	270
Mozzarella, part-skim	185
Cottage Cheese (½ cup)	
Calcium fortified cottage cheese	300
Ice Cream	
Regular, ½ cup	90
Low fat, ½ cup	100
Frozen Yogurt	
Low fat, ½ cup	100
Beans, dried, cooked, 1 cup	90
Salmon, with bones, 3 ounces	205
Tofu, calcium sulfate, ½ cup	435
Spinach, fresh cooked	244
Turnip Greens, fresh cooked, 1 cup	100
Kale, fresh cooked	94
Broccoli, fresh cooked	75
Waffle, 7" diameter	180
Pancakes, (2) 4" diameter	115

* Low fat and nonfat varieties of foods are still good sources of calcium.

Shopping List
From: Practical Dietary Therapy Information. Guidelines on Overweight and Obesity. National Heart, Lung and Blood Institute.

<u>Dairy Case</u>
Low fat (1%) or skim milk
Low fat or reduced-fat cottage cheese
Fat free cottage cheese
Low fat or nonfat yogurt
Light or diet margarine (tub, squeeze or spray)
Reduced-fat or fat free sour cream
Fat free cream cheese
Eggs/egg substitutes

<u>Breads, Muffins, Rolls</u>
Bread, bagels, pita bread   English muffins
Yeast breads
(whole wheat, rye, pumpernickel, multi-grain, raisin)
Corn tortillas (not fried)   Low fat flour tortillas
Fat-free biscuit mix   Rice crackers
Challah

<u>Cereals, Crackers, Rice, Noodles, Pasta</u>
Plain cereal, dry or cooked
Saltines, soda crackers (low sodium or unsalted types)
Graham crackers   Other low fat crackers
Rice (brown, white)   Pasta (noodles, spaghetti)
Bulgur, couscous, kasha
Potato mixes (made without fat)
Rice mixes (made without fat)
Other
Wheat mixes   Tabouli grain salad
Hominy   Polenta
Polvillo   Hominy grits
Quinoa   Millet
Aramanth   Oatmeal

Meat Case
White meat chicken and turkey (skin off)
Fish (not battered)
Beef, round or sirloin
Extra lean ground beef such as ground round
Pork tenderloin
95% fat-free lunch meats or low-fat deli meats
Meat equivalents
        Tofu (or bean curd)
        Beans (see bean list)
        Eggs/egg substitutes (see dairy list)

Fruit (fresh, canned, and frozen)
Fresh fruit

Apples	Bananas	Peaches
Oranges	Pear	Grapes
Grapefruit	Apricot	Dried fruits
Cherries	Plums	Melons
Lemons	Limes	Plantains
Mango	Papaya	

Exotic Fresh Fruit

Kiwi	Olives	Figs
Quinces	Currants	Persimmons
Pomegranates	Anon	Caimito
Chirimoya	Mamey	Papayas
Zapote	Guava	Starfruit
Ugli fruit	Dried pickled plums	Litchee nuts
Winter melons		

Canned Fruit (in juice or water)
Canned pineappleApplesauce
Other canned fruit (mixed or plain)

Frozen Fruits (without added sugar)

Blueberries	Raspberries

100% fruit juice

Dried Fruit
Raisins/dried fruit (these tend to be higher in calories than fresh fruit)

Vegetables (fresh, canned, frozen)

Broccoli	Peas	Corn
Cauliflower	Squash	Green Beans

Green Leafy Vegetables

Spinach	Lettuce	Cabbage
Artichokes	Cucumber	Asparagus
Mushrooms	Carrots or celery	Onions
Potatoes	Tomatoes	Green peppers
Chilies	Tomatillos	

Canned Vegetables (low sodium or no salt added)
Canned tomatoes
Tomato sauce or pasta
Other canned vegetables
Canned vegetable soup, reduced sodium

Frozen Vegetables (without added fats)
Broccoli
Spinach
Mixed medley, etc.
Yucca

Exotic Frozen Vegetables

Okra	Dandelions	Eggplant
Grape leaves	Mustard greens	Kale
Leeks	Boniato	Chayote
Borenjena	Plantain	Cassava
Prickly pear cactus	Bamboo shoots	Chinese celery
Water chestnuts	Bok choy	Burdock root
Napa cabbage	Taro	Seaweed
Bean sprouts	Amaranth	Choy sum
Calabacita	Sea vegetables	Rubarb

Beans and legumes (if canned, no salt added)

Lentils	Black beans
Red beans (kidney beans)	Navy beans
Pinto beans	Blackeyed peas
Fava beans	Mung beans
Italian white beans	Canned bean soup
Great white northern beans	Chickpeas (garbanzo beans)

Dried beans, peas and lentils (without flavoring packets)

Baking Items

Flour	Sugar
Imitation butter (flakes or buds)	Nonstick cooking spray
Canned evaporated milk, fat free	Nonfat dry milk powder
Cocoa powder, unsweetened	Baking powder
Baking soda	
Cornstarch	Unflavored gelatin
Angel food cake mix	Other low fat mixes

Gelatin, any flavor (reduced calorie)
Pudding mixes (reduced calorie)

Frozen Foods

Fish fillets, unbreaded	Egg subsitute
Fruits (no sugar added)	Vegetables (plain)

100% fruit juices (no sugar added)

Condiments, Sauces, Seasonings, and Spreads

Low fat or non fat salad dressings	Mustard (Dijon, etc)
Catsup	Barbecue sauce
Other low fat sauces	Jam, jelly or honey
Spices	Flavored vinegars
Hoisin sauce, plum sauce	Salsa or picante sauce
Canned green chilies	Soy sauce (low sodium)

Bouillon cubes/granules (low sodium)

Beverages

No calorie drink mixes	Reduced calorie juices
Unsweetened iced tea	Carbonated water
Water	

Sweetness Equivalency Chart

You may substitute an artificial sweetener for the sugar in the recipes. This is an equivalency chart for EQUAL.

Sugar	Equal Packets	Equal for Spoonful	Equal For Recipes
2 teaspoons	1 packet	¼ teaspoon	2 teaspoons
1 tablespoon	1 ½ packets	½ teaspoon	1 tablespoon
¼ cup	6 packets	1 ¾ teaspoons	¼ cup
⅓ cup	8 packets	2 ½ teaspoons	⅓ cup
½ cup	12 packets	3 ½ teaspoons	½ cup
¾ cup	18 packets	5 ½ teaspoons	¾ cup
1 cup	24 packets	7 ¼ teaspoons	1 cup

Eating Out

Here are the National Heart, Lung and Blood Institute Obesity
Guidelines for healthy eating out from the National Institutes of Health.
ASK! Will the restaurant:
- Serve margarine rather than butter with the meal?
- Serve skim milk rather than whole milk or cream?
- Trim visible fat from poultry or meat?
- Leave all butter, gravy or sauces off a dish?
- Serve salad dressing on the side?
- Accommodate special requests?
- Use less cooking oil when cooking?

ACT! Select foods that are:

Steamed	Garden Fresh	Broiled
Baked	Roasted	Poached
Lightly sautéed	Stir-fried	

Eating Healthy With Ethnic Food

The new National Heart, Lung, and Blood Institute Obesity Guidelines
recommend trying different ethnic cuisines to give yourself a taste treat
while losing weight. Many ethnic cuisines offer lots of low fat, low
calorie choices. Here's what to look for when making your selection.

Chinese

Steamed	Jum (poached)	Kow (roasted)
Shu (barbecued)	Steamed rice	MSG free

Italian

Red sauces	Primavera (no cream)
Piccata (lemon)	Sun-dried tomatoes
Crushed tomatoes	Lightly sautéed
Grilled	

Mexican

Spicy chicken	Rice & Black Beans
Salsa or picante	Soft corn tortillas

Tips For Getting More Calcium Into Your Diet

1. Add dry skim milk powder to hot cooked cereals.
2. Add dry skim milk powder to chili, meatloaf, soups and stews.
3. Add a slice of cheese to a sandwich.
4. Try using tofu instead of meat in stir-fry recipes
5. Switch from butter to fat free cream cheese on bread.
6. Sprinkle Parmesan cheese on vegetables. Much better than slathering them with butter and salt.
7. Toss a few cubes of your favorite reduced fat cheese into your soup just before serving.
8. Start buying the darker green varieties of lettuce, like Romaine. The darker the leaf, the bigger the calcium punch.
9. Love to put up your own home pickles? Make the brine with calcium chloride instead of sodium chloride (table salt).
10. Toss ¼ cup powdered nonfat dry milk into your baking recipes. It won't alter the recipe and will add extra calcium to your favorite treats.
11. Use your leftover vegetable cooking water in soups and stews, retaining the leached calcium.
12. Make your own soup with soup bones and a dash of vinegar in the cooking water to release the calcium stored in soup bones.
13. Look for mineral water with the highest calcium content.
14. Look for low sodium products in your grocery store and use them. Reducing the salt in your diet helps your calcium levels.
15. Look for calcium enriched products and use them wherever possible to boost your calcium levels.
16. Mix salsa with nonfat yogurt and use as a topping on baked potatoes, or as a dip for your favorite veggies.
17. Add evaporated skim milk to sauces, puddings and cream soups, right out of the can for a creamier taste.
18. Add a little yogurt to your mashed potatoes.
19. Add powdered skim milk to your pancake batter.
20. Add powdered skim milk to your mashed potatoes…or toss in a ¼ cup of Parmesan cheese.
21. Blend together a little fresh or frozen fruit and nonfat yogurt. A great topping for fresh fruit, pudding, cake, jello.

22. Stir dry skim milk powder into your coffee—tastes creamy and rich and adds major calcium.
23. Keep some buttermilk on hand. It can be substituted for milk in any recipe. Just add ½ teaspoon baking powder for each cup you substitute.
24. Add a little chopped parsley to your daily salad.
25. Snack on a handful nuts—better than salty, fatty snacks.
26. Discover the sweetness and calcium goodness of dried fruits, such as dates, figs, and raisins.
27. Get a can of nonfat evaporated milk. Pour it into a shallow dish. Put it into the freezer until ice crystals form around the edge. Transfer to a chilled bowl. Beat with chilled beaters until fluffy. Add a couple of teaspoons of confectioner's sugar. Beat again. Makes a great topping for your favorite dessert.
28. Switch from mayonnaise and sour cream, to plain, nonfat yogurt in dressings and dips.
29. Toss a handful of frozen okra, beet greens or kale into canned vegetable soup.
30. Top your veggies with shredded cheese and throw under the broiler for a minute.

Calcium Content 21-Days

Diet Day	Food-derived calcium in mg
Week 1-Day 1	1410
Week 1-Day 2	822
Week 1-Day 3	1006
Week 1-Day 4	901
Week 1-Day 5	1369
Week 1-Day 6	1470
Week 1-Day 7	1080
Week 2-Day 8	1798
Week 2-Day 9	1461
Week 2-Day 10	999
Week 2-Day 11	1371
Week 2-Day 12	1782
Week 2-Day 13	1774
Week 2-Day 14	1429
Week 3-Day 15	1517
Week 3-Day 16	1589
Week 3-Day 17	1711
Week 3-Day 18	1390
Week 3-Day 19	1735
Week 3-Day 20	819
Week 3-Day 21	1051

Calcium Content Non-Dairy 7-Days

Diet Day	Food-derived calcium in mg
Week 1-Day 1	682
Week 1-Day 2	463
Week 1-Day 3	899
Week 1-Day 4	948
Week 1-Day 5	550
Week 1-Day 6	684
Week 1-Day 7	851

Note: Calcium values may change depending on brands, freshness and other factors. These values are approximate.

Organizations

American Dietetic Association
216 West Jackson Blvd.
Chicago, IL 60606
www.eatright.org

American College of Obstetricians and Gynecologists
Resource Center
409 12th Street, S.W.
Washington, D.C. 20024
www.acog.org

American Academy for the Advancement of Medicine
23121 Verdugo Drive
Suite 204
Laguna Hills, CA 92653
www.acam.org

American Heart Association
7320 Greenville Avenue
Dallas, TX 75231
www.americanheart.org

American Association of Retired Persons (AARP)
601 E. Street, N.W.
Washington, D.C. 20049
www.aarp.org

American Diabetes Association
1660 Duke St.
Alexandria, VA 22314
www.diabetes.org

National Cancer Institute
9000 Rockville Pike
Building 31, Room 10A24
Bethesda, MD 20892
www.cancer.gov

Food and Drug Administration
5600 Fishers Lane
Rockville, MD 20857
Phone: 301-443-3170
www.fda.gov

National Osteoporosis Foundation
1150 17th Street, N.W.
Suite 500
Washington, D.C. 20036
www.nof.org

National Institute on Aging
P.O. Box 8057
Gaithersburg, MD 20898
www.nia.nih.gov

National Institutes of Health
Federal Building
Room 6C12
Bethesda, MD 20892
www.nih.gov

Research

American Journal of Clinical Nutrition, Effect of lifestyle intervention on bone mineral density in pre-menopausal women: A randomized trial. 70: 97-103, 1999.

American Diabetes Association.

American Heart Association.

Position of the American Dietetic Association: Weight Management. American Dietetic Association.

Ambrozy SL, et al. Effects of dietary calcium on blood pressure, vascular reactivity and vascular smooth muscle calcium efflux rate in Zucker rats. *American Journal of Hypertension.* 1991 Jul;4(7 pt 1):592-6

Buchowski, MS, et.al. Dietary calcium Intake in lactose maldigesting intolerant and African-American women. *Journal of American College of Nutrition.* 2002; 21: 47-54.

Carruth, BR, et al. The role of dietary calcium and other nutrients in moderating body fat in preschool children. *International Journal of Obestiy.* 2001; 25: 559-566.

Centers for Disease Control.

Cifuentes M et al. Energy restriction reduces fractional absorption in mature obese and lean rats. *Journal Nutrition* 2002. Sept;132(9):2660-6.

Compson JE. Vitamin D deficiency: time for action. Evidence supports routine supplementation for elderly people and others at risk. *BMJ* 1998 Nov 28;317(7171):1466-7

Davies, KM, et al. Calcium intake and body weight. *Journal of Clinical Endocrinology & Metabolism.* 2000; 85: 2-5.

Fleming, KH, Heimbach JT. Consumption of calcium in the U.S. food sources and intake levels. Journal of Nutrition. 1994 Aug;124(8 Suppl): 1426S-1430S.

Garland CF, et al. Calcium and vitamin D. Their potential roles in colon cancer and breast cancer prevention. *Ann N Y Academy of Science.* 1999;899:107-19.

Heaney RP et al. Calcium and weight: clinical studies. *Journal of the American College of Nutrition* 2002. Apr;21(2):152S-155S.

Heaney RP. Normalizing calcium intake: projected population effects for body weight. *J Nutr* 2003 Jan;133(1):268S-270S.

Kamycheva E et al. Intakes of calcium and vitamin d predict body mass index in the population of Northern Norway. *Journal of Nutrition* 2003 Jan;133(1):102-6

Levy J, et al. Role of cellular calcium metabolism in abnormal glucose metabolism and diabetic hypertension. *American Journal of Medicine.* 1989 Dec 8;87(6A):7S-16S. Review.

Melanson EL et al. Relation between calcium intake and fat oxidation in adult humans. *International Journal of Obesity Related Metabolic Disorders* 2003 Feb;27(2):196-203.

National Dairy Council.

National Institute of Child Health and Human Development (NICHD).

National Institute of Diabetes and Digestive and Kidney Diseases of the National Institutes of Health.

Ostman EM et al. Inconsistency between glycemic and insulinemic responses to regular and fermented milk products. *American Journal of Clinical Nutrition.* 2001;74:96-100.

Parikh SJ et al Calcium intake and adiposity. *American Journal of Clinical Nutrition* 2003 Feb;77(2):281-7.

Pereira MA, et al. Dairy consumption, obesity, and the insulin resistance syndrome in young adults: the CARDIA Study. *JAMA.* 2002;287:2081-2089.

Reusch JE et al. Regulation of GLUT-4 phosphorylation by intracellular calcium in adipocytes. *Endocrinology.* 1991;129:3269-3273.

Shi, H, et al. Effects of dietary calcium on adipocyte lipid metabolism and body weight regularion in energy-restricted mice. The University of Tennessee, Knoxville, TN. *Experimental Biology* 2000.

Shi, H., et al. Role of intracellular calcium in human adipocyte differentiation. *Obesity Research* 1999. Nov:7:50. (Suppl. 1: abstr. 083). *Physiol Genomics.* 2000 Aug 9;3(2): 75-82.

Tanasecu, M, et al. Biobehavioral Factors are associated with obesity in Puerto Rican children. Journal of Nutrition. 2000; 130: 1734-1742.

Teegarden D. Calcium intake and reduction in weight or fat mass. *J Nutrition* 2003 Jan;133(1):249S-251S.

Teegarden D, et al. Dairy calcium is related to changes in body composition during a two-year exercise intervention in young women. *Journal of the American College of Nutrition.* 2000; 19(6): 754-60.

Teegarden D, et al. Calcium intake relates to change in body weight in young women. *Experimental Biology* 1999.

Vaskonen T, et al. Effects of calcium and plant sterols on serum lipids in obese Zucker rats on a low-fat diet. *British Journal of Nutrition.* 2002 Mar;87(3): 239-45.

Xue B, et al. Mechanism of intracellular calcium inhibition of lipolysis in human adipocytes. The University of Tennessee, Knoxville, TN. *Experimental Biology.* 2000.

Xue B, et al. The agouti gene product inhibits lipolysis in human adipocytes via Ca2-dependent mechanism. *FASEB Journal.* 1998 Oct; 12(13):1391-6.

Zemel, MB. Mechanisms of dairy modulation of adiposity. *Journal of Nutrition.* 133(1): 252S-256S, Jan 2003.

Zemel, MB, et al. Regulation of adiposity by dietary calcium. *Federation of American Societies for Experimental Biology (FASEB) Journal.* 2000; 14:1132-1138.

Zemel, MB, et al. Nutritional and endocrine modulation of intracellular calcium: implications in obesity, insulin resistance and hypertension. *Mol. Cell Biochem.* 1998 Nov;188(1-2):129-36.

Zemel, MB, et al. Agouti regulation of intracellular calcium: Role in the insulin resistance of viable yellow mice. *Procedures of the National Academy of Science.* 1995 May 23;92(11):4733-7

Note: All nutritional values for recipes were developed with the aid of Master Cook by Sierra.

To Order Or For More Information

Please write to:
The Calcium Diet
830-13 A1A North
Ponte Vedra Beach, Florida 32082

Or Call Toll-Free
1-866-3-CALCIUM or 1-888-7-SKINNY

Or visit
www.thecalciumdiet.com or www.skinny.com

To Get Your FREE Offer

Call 1-866-3-CALCIUM

Or Visit Our Website

www.TheCalciumDiet.com

Our Free Offers Change So Please Check.
You will be asked to send proof of purchase and a cashiers check or money order for $8.99 shipping & handling.

By Mail: Please send proof of purchase (original bookstore receipt) and your name, address, phone number and email
PLUS $8.99 s/h to
FREE Calcium Diet Offer
The Calcium Diet
830-13 A1A North
Ponte Vedra Beach, FL 32082

By Phone:
Please call 1-866-3-CALCIUM or 1-888-7-SKINNY

On Line:
Please log on to www.thecalciumdiet.com or
www.skinny.com and select the button for FREE
CALCIUM DIET OFFER. Please follow the instructions.

Please note: FREE offers are available only while supplies last and may be changed or terminated at any time. You may be asked to pay a shipping and handling fee. Please allow 6 to 12 weeks for delivery. Publisher reserves the right to change or cancel the offer at any time without further notice.